T0199283

The Guidebook for Patient Counseling

THE GUIDEBOOK FOR
PATIENT
COUNSELING

HARVEY M. RAPPAPORT, Ph.D.
*Head of the Pharmacy Administration Division &
Associate Professor of Pharmacy and
Health Care Administration
Northeast Louisiana University
School of Pharmacy*

KELLY S. STRAKER, PharmD.
*Assistant Professor, Northeast Louisiana University
School of Pharmacy & Clinical Coordinator
Glenwood Regional Medical Center*

TRACY S. HUNTER, Ph.D.
*Associate Professor, Northeast Louisiana University
School of Pharmacy*

JOSEPH F. ROY, J.D.
*Professor, Northeast Louisiana University
School of Pharmacy*

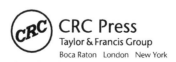

CRC Press
Taylor & Francis Group
Boca Raton London New York

CRC Press is an imprint of the
Taylor & Francis Group, an informa business

Reprinted 2010 by CRC Press

CRC Press
6000 Broken Sound Parkway, NW
Suite 300, Boca Raton, FL 33487
270 Madison Avenue
New York, NY 10016
2 Park Square, Milton Park
Abingdon, Oxon OX14 4RN, UK

The Guidebook for Patient Counseling

a **TECHNOMIC**ᵏ publication

Published in the Western Hemisphere by
Technomic Publishing Company, Inc.
851 New Holland Avenue, Box 3535
Lancaster, Pennsylvania 17604 U.S.A.

Distributed in the Rest of the World by
Technomic Publishing AG
Missionsstrasse 44
CH-4055 Basel, Switzerland

10 9 8 7 6 5 4 3 2

Main entry under title:
    The Guidebook for Patient Counseling

A Technomic Publishing Company book
Bibliography
Includes index p. 91

Library of Congress Catalog Card No. 93-79389
ISBN No. 1-56676-089-5

Patient medication counseling by pharmacists is coming of age. Whether mandated by professional standards of practice or by state and federal law, pharmacists may no longer have the luxury of ignoring their obligations to do so. Yet this may still be a palatable prescription. Reducing medication costs is the driving force behind this movement, and, if pharmacist counseling services are shown to be cost-effective, then pharmacists may be compensated on a scale far more than the mere sale of a product.

While specific details are still to be interpreted, the implications of the new state and federal laws requiring patient counseling are clear. The Omnibus Budget Reconciliation Act of 1990 (OBRA'90) mandates patient counseling, drug utilization review, and patient profiles, etc. State boards of pharmacy are rapidly adding counseling activities to licensing requirements, dramatically increasing pharmacists' responsibilities beyond the dispensing of prescriptions. There can be no doubt that these "official" new duties are here to stay.

This book is designed to assist practitioners to fully comply with the professional and legal requirements for patient counseling. It allows the pharmacist to choose the level at which to proceed. Those who wish to develop a practice based upon strong counseling will find this to be a complete and effective resource. Others can use it to satisfy minimal legal counseling requirements. More importantly, this is not intended to be a textbook to be briefly scanned and then put on the shelf. It is to be read and carried in your pocket instead. We have tried to develop a practical guide for pharmacists who wish to counsel and those who feel that they must do so. This book presents the skills pharmacists need to step out from behind the counter and counsel patients. These counseling skills can then be cultivated with study and practice. The book is meant to be used by any pharmacist practicing in any type of community pharmacy practice setting.

Finally, the book will acquaint the practitioner with: (1) a practical understanding of the nature of patient counseling, i.e., patient attitude and behavior, effect on compliance, the pharmacist-patient relationship, liability implications; (2) the skills required to effectively counsel, i.e., communications skills, using the prescription label, patient profiles and support personnel; and (3) realistic patient counseling scenarios that are easily adaptable to actual patient counseling situations.

Harvey M. Rappaport
Kelly S. Straker
Tracy S. Hunter
Joseph F. Roy

ACKNOWLEDGEMENTS

We would like to acknowledge the help of several people who afforded us the opportunity to complete this text. In particular, we appreciate the professional courtesy of our Australian colleague Dr. Michael Ortiz by permitting us to "glean" through his work. A great deal of thanks goes to the Pharmacy Administration graduate program at Northeast Louisiana University and its motivated students, most specifically Mr. Rajender Aparasu whose computer savvy spared us from any number of technical difficulties. And finally, a special nod goes to Ms. Beverly Gregory for her invaluable secretarial skills and patience.

CHAPTER 1

The Pharmacist-Patient Relationship

The willingness or desire to counsel and advise patients about their medication needs may be rooted in the pharmacist-patient relationship. An understanding of the nature of this relationship can be instrumental in motivating pharmacists to use their patient counseling skills.

But what is the pharmacist-patient relationship? Ethical and professional considerations suggest that it be described as an effective interaction between two parties having shared responsibility for health-care outcomes. Thus, the pharmacist would be expected to fill the medication needs of the patient and provide a full measure of professional ability as a health-care practitioner, while the patient would respond with full medication compliance. This view of the pharmacist-patient relationship appears consistent with the current practice philosophy known as ''pharmaceutical care.''

Pharmaceutical care has been defined as ''the responsible provision of drug therapy for the purpose of achieving definite outcomes that improve the patient's quality of life.'' The possible outcomes include: (1) cure a disease, (2) eliminate or reduce the patient's symptoms, (3) arrest or slow a disease's progress, and (4) prevent a disease or symptoms of a disease. Thus, under pharmaceutical care as well, the pharmacist provides pharmaceutical expertise in exchange for a patient's medication compliance.

The pharmacist-patient relationship, under pharmaceutical care, is fundamentally grounded in the concept of the professional covenant. A covenant is a mutual exchange of benefits in which the patient grants authority and trust to the provider (pharmacist) and the provider promises competence and commitment to the patient. The covenant relies on mutual trust, respect, and application of ethical values. Professionals add to this commitment, a large body of knowledge and acceptance of responsibility for their patient's welfare.

The proposed Code of Ethics for pharmacists being drafted by the

1

Using the following scale. please indicate *your response* for each statement by circling the appropriate number provided. *Please be completely honest in your response.*

	Strongly Disagree 1	Disagree 2	Undecided 3	Agree 4	Strongly Agree 5
	SD	D	U	A	SA
1. You are primarily interested in providing services to your patients.	1	2	3	4	5
2. You are becoming more involved in the selection of suppliers of the medications you dispense.	1	2	3	4	5
3. You do not rely on practice standards established by pharmaceutical organizations.	1	2	3	4	5
4. Filling a prescription correctly is not the most important part of your pharmacist-patient relationship.	1	2	3	4	5
5. You counsel patients even if not legally required to do so.	1	2	3	4	5
6. You are involved primarily in a business in which medications are dispensed in return for monetary compensation.	1	2	3	4	5
7. You are committed to your patients to practice competently.	1	2	3	4	5
8. Your work as a pharmacist is best judged by other pharmacists.	1	2	3	4	5
9. You practice pharmacy better with limited regulation from outside the profession.	1	2	3	4	5

FIGURE 1.1. The pharmacist-patient relationship test

Strongly Disagree 1	Disagree 2	Undecided 3	Agree 4	Strongly Agree 5
	SD	D	U	A	SA

		SD	D	U	A	SA
10.	You routinely monitor your patients for adverse reactions and interactions.	1	2	3	4	5
11.	You are capable of safely and effectively *prescribing* certain prescription-only drugs.	1	2	3	4	5
12.	Informed consent is less important than mutual trust in the pharmacist-patient relationship.	1	2	3	4	5
13.	You put your business concerns ahead of your professional obligations.	1	2	3	4	5
14.	You work first for the patient's best interest even when it is in conflict with your own.	1	2	3	4	5
15.	You practice your profession based on a continuing commitment to help others.	1	2	3	4	5
16.	You counsel even if you are not compensated for doing so.	1	2	3	4	5
17.	Trust is the most important element in your pharmacist-patient relationship.	1	2	3	4	5
18.	Your *primary* goal as a pharmacist is not to make money.	1	2	3	4	5
19.	You routinely monitor patients to maximize compliance with drug therapy.	1	2	3	4	5

FIGURE 1.1 (continued). The pharmacist-patient relationship test

Strongly Disagree 1	Disagree 2	Undecided 3	Agree 4	Strongly Agree 5
		SD D	U	A SA
20. A patient's medication profile is more accurate when a single pharmacy is used for all medication needs, *even if it isn't yours*.		1 2	3	4 5

When you are done, add all the numbers circled and divide by 20. This will give your average attitude score. The reliability of the test suggests that your actual attitude towards the pharmacist-patient relationship will fall on the following continuum:

Professional Covenant	Contract Within Covenant	Professional Contract

5 - - - - - - - - - - - 4 - - - - - - - - - - - 3 - - - - - - - - - - - 2 - - - - - - - - - - - 1

However, you decide whether your score truly reflects your patient attitude and how your tendency to counsel patients is influenced by that attitude.

FIGURE 1.1 (continued). The pharmacist-patient relationship test

American Pharmaceutical Association suggests that the ethical conduct of pharmacists should be guided by a "covenantal relationship between the patient and the pharmacist." It further states that:

> Considering the patient-pharmacist relationship as a covenant means that each pharmacist has moral obligations in response to the gift of trust received from society. In return for this gift, the pharmacist promises to help individuals achieve optimum benefit from their medications, to be committed to their welfare, and to maintain their trust.

However, many practitioners believe that they may be bound by a different pharmacist-patient relationship, that of the professional contract. This viewpoint suggests that, in addition to the professional characteristics, there is a mutually acceptable exchange of rights and obligations between practitioner (pharmacist) and patient. The heart of this relationship is informed consent rather than trust. Supporters argue that a contractual understanding of a therapeutic relationship encourages full respect for the dignity of the patient and full medication compliance. Yet both parties may tend to guard their own interests. Thus, the contract also provides for legal enforcement of the agreed-upon terms.

An interesting variation in the nature of the pharmacist-patient relationship is the idea that there is a contract within every professional covenant. Supporters of this view suggest that the professional pharmacist can fulfill all patient care commitments without neglecting one's own business interests. The stability of the business may even become the foundation for sustaining the pharmacist's ability to practice pharmaceutical care.

Is the professional covenant, professional contract, or some variation the most realistic assessment of the pharmacist-patient relationship? Which is most likely to act as a motivating force in encouraging pharmacists to counsel patients under actual practice conditions? Perhaps a close look at the ways in which pharmacists perceive their own pharmacist-patient relationships can shed some light.

Accordingly, we have developed a test to assess a pharmacist's attitude towards the pharmacist-patient relationship. "Attitude" signifies the way one sees relationships in the environment based upon past experiences. What attitude do you have towards your patients in your practice setting? Depending on the nature of your relations with your patients, this test could be used to measure that attitude (see Figure 1.1).

CHAPTER 2

State and Federal Statutes and Regulations Concerning Patient Counseling

OBRA`90 is an acronym for the Omnibus Budget Reconciliation Act of 1990. As is evident from the term "Budget," this Act consists of fiscal, budgetary and related provisions. "Omnibus" indicates that it is a mosaic of legislation, affecting many areas of federal law. Although it would be more proper to refer to the specific part of the Act which concerns pharmacists and patient counseling, the acronym for the entire Act has become synonymous with this part and for ease of understanding, will be so designated in this chapter.

OBRA`90 consists of three major sections: pharmaceutical pricing and manufacturer rebate provisions; a drug use review program (DUR), of which patient counseling is a part; and demonstration projects. The pricing/rebate component went into effect shortly after enactment while the others were not to become effective until January 1, 1993.

The primary effect of the DUR program is to improve the quality of care received by Medicaid beneficiaries by reducing their exposure to hazards resulting from the inappropriate prescribing, dispensing and use of prescription drugs. According to the Health Care and Financing Administration (HCFA), up to 30 percent of the prescriptions for several potential problem drugs were inappropriate.

The DUR program requirement had its genesis in the ill-fated Medicare Catastrophic Coverage Act of 1988, which contained the first provision for utilization review and patient counseling. The Act was repealed before becoming effective.

Subsequently, in 1990, two separate Senate bills were introduced but never passed. One was the Pharmaceutical Access and Prudent Purchasing Act (PAPPA), which would have established a national formulary under the auspices of a DUR Board. The other was the Patient Benefit Restoration Act (PBRA) which permitted an open formulary but also contained a

DUR/prior approval system. The PBRA was intended to restore some of the patient benefits lost by the repeal of the Medicare Catastrophic Coverage Act.

Because DUR programs are believed to improve the quality of pharmaceutical care while saving money, one was incorporated into OBRA`90. The Congressional Budget Office has estimated that annual combined federal and state savings will range from $10 to 40 million. As a result of more efficient and exact utilization of pharmaceutical therapy, a decrease in the number of prescriptions written and dispensed is expected.

Once OBRA`90 became law, its various provisions were merged into corresponding portions of the United States Code. The DUR program, with its patient counseling component, was added to Title XIX of the Social Security Act. This Title authorizes grants to those states electing to provide outpatient prescription drug coverage to needy individuals under their Medicaid plans. It is administered by HCFA, which published interim final regulations in the *Federal Register*, Vol. 57, No. 212 (November 2, 1992).

The DUR program is intended to improve the quality of pharmaceutical care by ensuring that prescriptions are appropriate, medically necessary and not likely to cause adverse medical results. "Adverse medical result" means a clinically significant undesirable effect, experienced by a patient, due to a course of drug therapy. "Appropriate and medically necessary" is defined as drug prescribing and dispensing in conformity with the predetermined standards developed or obtained by each state.

In order to qualify for federal financial participation, each electing state was to have its DUR program in operation by January 1, 1993. The program must consist of four components: prospective drug use review; retrospective drug use review; the application of predetermined standards; and an educational strategy.

Prospective DUR consists of a point-of-sale/distribution review of drug therapy before each prescription is filled or delivered, the maintenance of patient profiles and patient counseling. The review must include screening to identify potential drug therapy problems due to therapeutic duplication, drug-disease contraindication, adverse drug-drug interaction (including serious interactions with nonprescription or over-the-counter drugs), incorrect drug dosage, incorrect duration of drug treatment, drug-allergy interaction and clinical abuse/misuse.

These problems are defined as follows:

1. *Therapeutic duplication* – the prescribing and dispensing of two or more drugs from the same therapeutic class such that the combined daily dose puts the recipient at risk of an adverse medical result or incurs additional program costs without therapeutic benefit

2. *Drug-disease contraindication* – the potential for, or the occurrence of,

an undesirable alteration of the therapeutic effect of a given prescription because of the presence, in the patient for whom it is prescribed, of a disease condition or the potential for, or the occurrence of, an adverse effect of the drug on the patient's disease condition

3. *Adverse drug-drug interaction* — the potential for, or occurrence of, an adverse medical effect as a result of the recipient using two or more drugs together

4. *Incorrect drug dosage* — the dosage that lies outside the daily dosage range specified in the predetermined standards as necessary to achieve therapeutic benefit (Dosage range is the strength multiplied by the quantity dispensed divided by the day's supply.)

5. *Incorrect duration of drug treatment* — the number of days the prescribed therapy exceeds or falls short of the recommendations contained in the predetermined standards

6. *Drug-allergy interaction* — the significant potential for, or the occurrence of, an allergic reaction as a result of drug therapy

7. *Clinical abuse/misuse* — the occurrence of situations referred to in the definitions of abuse, gross overuse, overutilization, underutilization, incorrect dosage and incorrect duration
   a) Abuse: no definition provided in this section
   b) Gross overuse: repetitive overutilization without therapeutic benefit
   c) Overutilization: use of a drug in quantities or for durations that put the recipient at risk of an adverse medical result
   d) Underutilization: a drug is used by a recipient in insufficient quantity to achieve a desired therapeutic goal
   e) Incorrect dosage: refer to No. 4, above
   f) Incorrect duration: refer to No. 5, above

In addition to the screening provision of the prospective DUR program, the pharmacist must make a reasonable effort to obtain, record and maintain patient profiles of each Medicaid recipient. (See Chapter 7.) At a minimum, the profile must contain:

1. The name, address, telephone number and date of birth (or age) and gender of the patient

2. Individual medical history, where significant, including disease state(s), known allergies and drug reactions, and a comprehensive list of medications and relevant devices

3. Pharmacist comments relevant to the individual's drug therapy

HCFA suggests that the information developed from the patient profile be used to assist the pharmacist in the screening portion of the prospective

DUR process. Further, where appropriate, the pharmacist might consult a physician to obtain additional details.

The final phase of the prospective DUR process entails counseling of the patient. The pharmacist must *offer* to counsel the patient or caregiver about the prescription. At a minimum, the counseling must encompass an offer to discuss with the patient or caregiver certain matters that the pharmacist deems significant. The discussion must be in person where practicable; otherwise, by toll-free telephone service. It should include (in addition to those matters already deemed significant) at least the following:

1. The name and description of the medication
2. The dosage form, dosage, route of administration and use by the patient
3. Special directions and precautions for preparation, administration and use by the patient
4. Common severe side or adverse effects or interactions and therapeutic contraindications that may be encountered, including their avoidance, and the action required if they occur
5. Techniques for self-monitoring drug therapy
6. Proper storage
7. Prescription refill information
8. Action to be taken in the event of a missed dose

Although the pharmacist must *offer* to provide consultation, the patient or caregiver may refuse the offer. Apparently, counseling is the only element in the prospective DUR process which may be waived. Covered outpatient drugs exempt from OBRA'90 requirements include those dispensed by certain Health Maintenance Organizations (HMOs), those dispensed by a hospital using a drug formulary system and billing the state plan at a special cost, and those dispensed to residents of nursing facilities already in compliance with established drug regimen procedures.

In the Act, states are directed to make substantial changes to remain eligible for federal financial participation. Specifically pertaining to the prospective DUR process, states must provide pharmacies with detailed information as to what they must do to comply with the particular requirements. This includes guidelines on counseling, profiling and documentation of prospective DUR activities, as well as the development of counseling standards.

Most states have responded positively to these directives. When the interim final rule was being developed, HCFA estimated that 17 states already required an offer of counseling by pharmacists. By March, 1993, more than 80 percent of the states had made some effort to comply. The great majority implemented the prospective DUR criteria by administrative regulation, although several did so by statute and a few used both methods. HCFA has indicated either is acceptable.

A substantial majority of states have separated the prospective and retrospective DUR functions, leaving the latter with the agency or authority traditionally administering the Medicaid program and delegating the former to the pharmacy licensing or practice boards for implementation.

While OBRA'90 only covers Medicaid prescriptions, most states have extended the prospective DUR requirements to include all prescriptions. Nationally, in 1991, pharmacy payments under the Medicaid program were approximately $5.5 billion and comprised nearly 17 percent of the total revenue for prescription drugs. Undoubtedly, this has been an influential factor; however, pharmacy as a profession is to be commended for assuming a greater role in patient care.

Most states' guidelines materially follow the substantive prospective DUR criteria in OBRA'90; however, there are many differences in the details. Although most state statutes or regulations require an offer to counsel, the courts have strictly interpreted such provisions, holding them to be ''definitional'' rather than ''mandatory.'' (For an analysis of this distinction, refer to Chapter 3.)

The states differ in documentation standards, some specifying that a waiver of counseling should be in writing, while another, for example, states in its regulations that, '' The absence of any record of a failure to accept the pharmacist's offer to counsel shall be presumed to signify that such an offer was accepted and that such counseling was provided.''

Further, there are significant differences between the states in instructing the pharmacist on the steps to take should the screening review reveal one or more of the conditions for which the screening is performed. Some states' guidelines require that the physician be contacted, while others leave it to the pharmacist's discretion to resolve the problem.

Likewise, there are important variations between the states concerning whether the prospective DUR process should be performed for all prescriptions or whether distinctions may be made between new and refill prescriptions as well as between the types of refills.

Because each state is different, it is impossible to describe each one's particular provisions and compare and contrast them, and any such analysis would be of limited application. For the community pharmacist, it is recommended that familiarity with the substantive portions of OBRA'90 might serve as the best reference point. Then, learn those specific standards imposed by your state. Such preparation will accelerate development of your counseling techniques and enable you to render a higher standard of patient care.

CHAPTER 3

Liability and Other Legal Issues Affecting Patient Counseling

Liability is a legal or equitable obligation that arises when a duty owed is breached. If an injury results, the liable party may be called upon to compensate for the damage. This is known as negligence.

In the context of the pharmacist-patient relationship, for a pharmacist to be liable to a patient, there must be a particular duty owed by the pharmacist to that patient. The pharmacist must then breach that duty by failing to meet a certain standard of care, and the substandard conduct must result in damages to the patient. Overall, this "pharmacist negligence" is characterized as *malpractice*, i.e., a professional's failure to exercise an accepted level of skill and knowledge, which results in harm to a client or patient.

The establishment of a particular duty owed to a patient is the most controversial aspect of pharmacy malpractice, and the recent widespread imposition of patient screening and counseling requirements have made an already complex situation even more complicated.

Historically, pharmacists have been held to the strictest, highest standard in their dispensing functions. Cases and commentaries from the nineteenth century have set forth a standard for druggists and apothecaries as one where they must not only be skillful, but also exceedingly cautious and prudent. It should be remembered that pharmacists routinely prepared and dispensed harmful, even poisonous, substances, so the various courts consistently noted that people trust their very lives to the knowledge, care and prudence of druggists. The care required should properly and reasonably be proportional to the danger involved.

Most reported cases concerned dispensing errors in one form or another, although in the 1930s there were a few instances where courts somewhat hesitatingly found expanded duties to patients. In a 1934 Louisiana case, a pharmacist did not comply with a state health regulation requiring the obtaining and entering of certain patient data in the poison register. Carbolic

13

acid was dispensed to an " imbecile," a twenty-one-year-old woman unable to apprehend or appreciate the product's potentially lethal nature. She drank it and died. Although in its decision the state supreme court used the term "negligent dispensing," its core holding was that the pharmacist breached a duty to the patient in not acquiring the information that would have revealed the patient's mental deficit. Essentially, the pharmacist was responsible for ascertaining the patient's competence to use an otherwise properly prepared, dispensed and labeled product.

In a Kansas case adjudicated that same year, the pharmacist recommended that a patient suffering from a skin disorder substitute a nonprescription ointment for a prescription one already being used; however, the pharmacist did not inform the patient that the two products could adversely interact. When this occurred, and skin damage resulted, the pharmacist told the patient to continue using only the nonprescription item, which aggravated the condition. In its decision holding the pharmacist liable, the court found that when recommending a medication, a pharmacist is held to the highest degree of care in advising of harmful effects. As in the Louisiana case, the Kansas court indicated there were circumstances where a pharmacist could owe a duty which extended beyond accurate dispensing to ascertaining proper use.

The value of these cases lies in their implications of pharmacists' expanded responsibilities and the courts' tentative explorations toward recognition; however, because of the unusual facts presented in each, their applications are very limited. Neither involved physicians' prescriptions; thus, the question of a pharmacist's liability to a patient for harm when accurately filling and dispensing such a prescription was not addressed.

Well through the 1970s, virtually all instances where a pharmacist was found liable for damages involved various types of dispensing errors; and, from the 1950s onward, those cases where a pharmacist failed to accurately interpret, fill or otherwise execute a physician's prescription began to dominate.

The courts came to regard the pharmacist as a sort of " super-technician," having a near-absolute duty of error-free disper :ng, but owing nothing else to the patient. This differentiated pharmacists from other professionals, who are not held to perfection but to a level of skill and knowledge commonly possessed by other licensed practitioners in similar communities.

During the 1980s, a new view of pharmacists began to emerge. Approximately two dozen cases were reported where pharmacists were sued, not for negligent dispensing, but for failing to warn patients of the dangerous properties of certain medications. The allegations ranged from failing to advise of potentially harmful interactions of and reactions to particular drugs to not alerting patients to their addictive qualities. The theory of liability underpinning these suits was that the pharmacist breached a duty to warn, i.e., to provide information. Conceptually, the pharmacist, as a skilled and knowledgeable practitioner, knew, or should have known, of a reasonably foreseeable risk of harm to the patient from using the particular drug and, therefore, owed a duty to warn of the danger.

In response to these lawsuits, the pharmacists generally asserted they owed no such duty; their only responsibility was to accurately fill and dispense the physicians' prescriptions. It was the doctor who should advise about medications and their potentially harmful effects. For the pharmacists to also discuss drugs with patients would interfere with the doctor-patient relationship.

Most courts agreed with the pharmacists' arguments and did not favor examining the doctor-patient relationship in a broader health-care environment; nor did they favor analyzing it in conjunction with any pharmacist-patient relationship. It seemed wise public policy to affix responsibility directly on the physician.

It is accepted legal theory that some products are designed and manufactured that are ''unavoidably unsafe'' for their intended and ordinary use; however, their benefits are too great to deny them to the consumer. Those products, such as drugs, may be marketed but only with accompanying proper and adequate warnings and directions. Under these conditions, when a manufacturer of a particular drug provides the required information to a physician who then prescribes that drug for a patient, the manufacturer is usually not liable for any damages the patient may sustain as a result of using the drug. The physician is the ''informed intermediary'' between the manufacturer and the patient.

Pharmacists successfully raised the informed intermediary defense even though it had only previously been applied to pharmaceutical manufacturers. The courts were receptive because it seemed to reinforce the completeness of the doctor-patient relationship. Conversely, any possibility of recognizing an independent pharmacist-patient relationship was diminished. Thus, as a general rule, pharmacists owed no duty to warn of possible adverse effects of medication usage.

Notable exceptions to this trend were 1982 New York and 1990 Tennessee cases. In the former, *Hand v. Krakowski*, during a ten-month period, a pharmacist dispensed 728 units of ''opiate-type'' (but otherwise unidentified) psychotropic drugs, presumably in accordance with valid prescriptions, to a patient who was identified in the pharmacist's records as a ''known alcoholic.'' The patient died allegedly as a result of the drug and alcohol combination. The court found the pharmacist knew, or should have known, that the drugs were ''contraindicated'' with alcohol and, therefore, were extremely dangerous to the patient's well-being. Under such circumstances. ". . . The dispensing druggist may have had a duty to warn decedent of the grave danger involved and to inquire of the prescribing doctors if such drugs should not be discontinued."

The latter, Tennessee case, *Dooley v. Everett*, involved the issue of whether a pharmacist had a duty to warn a patient, the physician, or both of the potential interaction between two different prescription drugs, written by the same physician on two different days for a three-year-old child. The drugs were theophylline and erythromycin; all prescriptions were accurately dispensed. The child suffered cerebral seizures. In its decision, the court refused to extend the learned intermediary doctrine to the (pharmacist's) patient and focused on whether the scope of duty owed by the pharmacist includes a duty to warn. It recognized that, "The pharmacist is a professional who has a duty to his customer to exercise the standard of care required by the pharmacy profession in the same or similar communities as the community in which he practices his profession."

Both *Hand* and *Dooley* concerned prescriptions that were valid on their faces but that the courts believed should have been questioned by the pharmacists. Once doubts were raised, the duty was attached to warn the patient, inquire of the physician, or both.

In two cases from this same period, pharmacists were presented with prescriptions that contained inadequate directions or incorrect dosages; in other words, they were questionable on their faces. In the 1986 Pennsylvania case of *Riff v. Morgan Pharmacy*, Cafergot® suppositories were prescribed with written instructions to insert one every four hours for headache, with no notations authorizing refills. The pharmacist dispensed as written, typing the same instruction on the label. Not experiencing relief, the patient obtained refills from the pharmacist and used as indicated but greatly exceeded the accepted maximum dosages of two per attack, with a limit of five in any week. The patient suffered permanent injuries to her foot from decreased circulation and nerve damage. The court found the physician and the pharmacist liable; the latter because of breach of duty by ". . . failing to warn the patient or notify the prescribing physician of the obvious inadequacies appearing on the face of the prescription which created a substantial risk of serious harm to the plaintiff." Its reasoning emphasized that the pharmacist is a professional who owes a duty to the patient and has more responsibility than to be a ". . . shipping clerk who must dutifully and *unquestionably* obey the written orders of omniscient physicians."

In the 1987 Louisiana case of *Hendricks v. Charity Hospital of New Orleans, et al.*, a pharmacist was presented with a prescription that specified an overdosage of Dilantin®. The pharmacist sent the patient back to the physician, who confirmed the dosage. When the patient returned to the drugstore and advised of the validation, the pharmacist unsuccessfully tried to contact the physician. Because the patient needed to begin therapy, the pharmacist dispensed the medication with the incorrect instructions and a note that the patient should consult the physician about dosage on the label. Soon, the patient suffered Dilantin® toxicity. At issue was whether the pharmacist breached a duty ``. . . to take some reasonable steps to locate plaintiff and warn him of the dangerous position he was in.`` The court concluded that, although a close call, the pharmacist's conduct did not fall below the applicable standard and, hence, no duty was breached.

By the end of the 1980s, the overwhelming jurisprudential trend was against imposing a duty to warn on pharmacists, except in circumstances of obvious inadequacies in a prescription. Also during this period several state legislatures or pharmacy boards enacted or adopted statutes or regulations pertaining to patient counseling.

Counseling and warning are not the same. Warning is simply the provision of information; counseling involves the provision of information as well as assistance in usage. Thus, warning is a basic component of counseling and the threshold of the counseling process.

The first and most significant decision addressing the impact of counseling requirements was a 1989 Washington case, *McKee v. American Home Products Corporation*. For ten years, the patient received prescriptions for an amphetamine as weight loss therapy. The patient was 5'4" tall and at no time weighed more than 138 pounds. The pharmacist accurately filled the prescriptions and dispensed these drugs with no advice or warning to the patient about potentially hazardous side effects. Suit was filed alleging injuries as a result of addiction.

Washington pharmacy practice statutes provided for the maintenance of patient medication records ``. . . which may include information on `allergies, idiosyncracies or chronic conditions which may relate to drug utilization.`` `` In defining the ``practice of pharmacy,`` the statutory provisions included the practice of and responsibility for ``. . . the monitoring of drug therapy . . .`` and ``. . . the providing of information on legend drugs which may include, but is not limited to, the advising of therapeutic values, hazards, and the uses of drugs and devices.``

In its decision, the state supreme court split 5−4, dismissing the suit on technical grounds relating to the sufficiency of an affidavit in a summary procedure. Then, it addressed these other issues because of their importance and public interest.

It found the patient counseling and drug monitoring provisions to be ``definitional,`` not mandatory; and, thus, no duty was imposed on pharmacists to warn patients by virtue of the statutes. Further, the court determined that the monitoring requirement pertained to institutional, not community, pharmacists.

Next, the court analyzed current jurisprudence, distinguishing the *Hand* and *Riff* cases as instances of patent errors in a prescription for which the pharmacist has a duty to be alert and to take corrective action. It adopted the informed intermediary doctrine, noting that a pharmacist has neither the medical education or knowledge of the patient's medical history to justify an "intrusion" into the physician-patient relationship. The majority concluded that a pharmacist has a duty to be alert for clear errors or mistakes in the prescription but not to question a physician's judgment concerning the propriety of a prescription or to warn of the hazardous side effects associated with a drug.

Although it would seem that *McKee*, as dicta and as the product of a seriously divided court, would have limited precedential value, two subsequent decisions have substantially followed its reasoning. The first was a 1991 Kansas case, *Nichols v. Central Merchandise, Inc.*, which also discussed a counseling provision. Pharmacy practice regulations stated, in pertinent part, that a pharmacist's duties included ". . . initiating oral patient consultation on new prescriptions as a matter of routine to encourage proper patient drug utilization and administration." The court held that warning labels satisfied the requirement of encouraging proper utilization and administration; and, otherwise, because Kansas followed the learned intermediary doctrine, a pharmacist has no duty to warn.

The second and most recent treatment of patient counseling functions was a 1992 Missouri case, *Kampe v. Howard Stark Professional Pharmacy, Inc.* At issue were statutes which defined the practice of pharmacy and relevantly included ". . . the interpretation and evaluation of prescription orders . . ." and ". . . consultation with patients and other health care practitioners about the safe and effective use of drugs and devices. . . ." Another section of the statute stated, "All pharmacists may provide pharmaceutical consultation and advice to persons concerning the safe and therapeutic use of prescription drugs."

The court first noted that the statutes were inapplicable to the matter before them because of their enactment date; however, if they were in effect, no duty to warn would be imposed. The provisions are "definitional," not mandatory, as evinced by the use of the permissive word "may" instead of "shall." "Use of 'may' in a statute implies alternate possibilities and that the ones to whom the power is granted, in this case pharmacists, have discretion in exercising that power."

These recent decisions, in conjunction with earlier rulings, indicate that courts will be reluctant to afford expansive interpretations to patient counseling and screening provisions and are not likely to recognize a duty to warn emanating from statutes or regulations unless clearly set forth. The pharmacists' responsibilities should be explicitly stated in imperative terms.

Nevertheless, most pharmacists will probably comply with their state directives and perform screening and counseling. Although a court may not recognize a legal duty, licensing or regulatory boards may certainly dictate practice requirements. A pharmacist who ignores practice standards because there is no legal duty might be in violation of professional rules or regulations. It would be little comfort to escape civil liability but be unable to practice.

When a pharmacist does undertake to warn or counsel, the standard of care to be used expands with the circumstances. In the 1986 North Carolina case of *Ferguson v. Williams*, the patient presented a prescription for Indocin®. While the prescription was being filled, the patient informed the pharmacist that he was allergic to aspirin, Percodan® and penicillin and asked if the prescribed drug was safe. Supposedly, the pharmacist responded affirmatively; the following day the patient died from an anaphylactic reaction. The court ruled that, ". . . Once a pharmacist is alerted to specific facts and he or she undertakes to advise a customer, the pharmacist has a duty to advise correctly."

As discussed earlier in this chapter, when dispensing advice, the pharmacist is not held to perfection, but to the standard in exercising skill and knowledge common to active practitioners in similar communities, under similar circumstances. This standard is one which other professionals have learned to meet. Overall, it has proved workable and fair. Pharmacists are too highly educated and trained to be relegated to the role of technicians. They possess a great deal of knowledge, skill and wisdom, which can benefit their patients and the entire health-care community.

CHAPTER 4

Overview of Communication Skills

The purpose of this chapter is to briefly review those communication skills and techniques that are the basis for providing effective patient counseling. Obstacles to effective counseling will also be addressed.

COMMUNICATION VS. INTERPERSONAL COMMUNICATION

Communication is the transfer of information meaningful to those involved. It occurs in forms ranging from face-to-face contact with attendant complex facial expressions and body movements, to simple written messages like auxiliary labels. It may be described as a process in which messages are generated and sent by one person and subsequently received and translated by another person.

A problem with communication is that although the intended message is generated by the sender, the meaning is generated within the receiver. That is, meaning is defined by the receiver's translation of the message, rather than the original intended message. Simply put, a message, a written instruction or a verbal instruction is not always translated to mean what was originally intended.

Interpersonal communication is an interactive process that involves an individual's effort to attain meaning and to respond accordingly. It involves the transmission and reception of verbal and non-verbal signs and symbols. Most of the emotional meaning of a message is contained in the non-verbal component. The nature of interpersonal communication between any two persons, such as a patient and a pharmacist, can be described as follows. Each person exists both in their own world, defined by their personal history and concepts of self, and that of the other person. As two people interact, each interprets the messages sent in a way that is consistent with his or her world, and then behaves based on these interpretations. The resulting behavior of either person then provides a potential meaning to the other. Unfortunately, this often results in misunderstanding.

LISTENING

The ability to listen effectively enhances the communication process. Unfortunately, most people are not good listeners. Effective listening is dependent on the attitude of the listener toward the speaker. When a patient respects a pharmacist and believes he or she will benefit from the communication, then the patient is more likely to listen to the pharmacist. Preoccupation with other matters may also stop individuals from listening to the pharmacist. Other barriers to effective listening include mentally arguing with comments made by the pharmacist before he or she finishes talking, a lack of interest in the message, and other negative reactions. The pharmacist will be more likely to listen for effective counseling by using certain phrases and questions. This will help keep the counseling session brief and effective through the creation of simple paraphrasing, useful ways to clarify important information, and active feedback (see Table 4.1).

NON-VERBAL COMMUNICATION

People convey meaning through silence and other non-verbal means of expression as well as through speech. Gestures, vocal intonations, facial expressions, and body posture are all forms of non-verbal communication. It is estimated that only about one-third of the meaning of a message is communicated by the words used. The remainder of the message is communicated non-verbally. A comparison of non-verbal messages with verbal communication is a powerful tool in identifying potential communication problems, particularly since most people are poor non-verbal liars. That is, patients tend to communicate non-verbally the part of the message that they wish least to communicate. Visual cues will lead to more accurate judgments regarding patient understanding of a message than what the patient tells you. Thus, non-verbal communication is a vital component in effective patient counseling. It is often easier for a pharmacist to listen to what the patient says and ignore the non-verbal components of the message, because the non-verbal message may suggest a problem that the pharmacist would prefer not to handle. For example, when patients are asked whether they understand how to take their medication, they may answer that they do, yet they will shake their head negatively from side to side. It is much easier for the pharmacist to respond to what the patient said, than follow up the negative, non-verbal message with further questions.

TABLE 4.1. Phrases and Questions That Aid Listening.

Paraphrase Openings

    Are you saying that . . . ?
    Do I understand you to mean . . . ?
    What I've heard so far is . . .
    Okay, so you've said that . . .
    Let me tell you what I am understanding.
    What I hear you saying is . . .
    Is what you are really saying . . . ?

Requests for Clarification

    What do you mean by . . . ?
    Who is it? Who is saying this?
    How do you know?
    What do you mean?
    I don't understand what you mean.
    Your reference is unfamiliar to me.
    I hear what you are saying, but you seem to feel another way.

Support Statements

    Would an example of that be . . . ?
    That's like when I . . . Is that what you're talking about?
    I've had that kind of experience too; why just last week . . .
    It made me feel . . . just as you've described.
    And did you . . . or?

Active Feedback

    I understand what you are saying (or I hear what you are saying).
    I see (or uh huh, really).
    Yes, that's how I found it to be.
    No, I don't feel that way, but let me hear why you do.
    I've not found that to be so, give me an example of . . . .

INTERACTIVE COMMUNICATION

Interactive communication establishes a dialogue with the patients. Patients are asked what they know about their treatment regimen or condition. The pharmacist can then fill in gaps in knowledge or correct misinformation. The interactive model is distinguished from the monologue approach by its style. To contrast the differences, think of styles of education. Interactive communication resembles a discussion, rather than an ordinary lecture. If you were to meet a research scientist at a reception and converse about her field, the tone and content of her description would adjust to the feedback that she received from you. If you attended one of her lectures, little feedback adjustment would be made. Interactive counseling is like the conversation. Feedback from the patient directs the pharmacist to focus the information. Remember, the desired result is not a patient who necessarily knows everything about diabetes, but one who will follow the prescribed treatment regimen and watch for warning signs. Additionally, you want the patient to feel open enough with you to ask ``dumb`` questions and to tell you about changes that may or may not be related to therapy. This is only possible when the patient feels that you care and understand by discussing therapy with her or him.

This conversation is particularly important when it comes to talking about sensitive issues. While sexual subject matter first comes to mind as an example of an area requiring tact and objectivity, there are less obvious and common ones. Such personal matters can include decreased functioning in the elderly, incontinence, discovery of a possible cancer, or change in bowel function.

Interactive patient counseling can also be described as a technique in which the pharmacist engages the patient in an exchange specifically to cover important practical matters about his or her medications. It verifies that the patient understands, fills in knowledge gaps, corrects misinformation and concludes with a brief summary. Interactive patient counseling furnishes several advantages to practitioners and patients. Rather than reciting a litany of ``Do's and Don'ts`` regarding the therapy, interactive counseling engages the patient in a brief discussion. The benefits of actively involving patients are: increased retention of key facts by patients, less time than using a monologue to recite facts, and, because it is personalized, a greater reward for both the patient and pharmacist.

EMPATHY

Empathy is the ability to see the world through another person's eyes, to enter into another's life and accurately perceive his or her current feelings. It is appropriate when the person simply needs someone to listen. If the patient feels that a practitioner is even trying to understand his feelings, he or she is much more receptive to advice. Empathy is a process to perceive and identify the surface and underlying feelings of the other person's statements, and respond in a manner that lets them know that you understand. It has three essential steps: facilitating, perceiving and responding.

Facilitating behavior shows attentiveness and establishes a comfortable and safe environment for patients to express their feelings. Perceiving involves seeking to identify and label the other's feelings. Responding is the activity that lets others know that you understand and are willing to hear more. The technique is meant to allow the pharmacist to effectively respond by trying to restate and reflect the patient's feelings. This is accomplished by repeating the essential content of what was heard with slightly different words. The phrases used in this approach include:

"It sounds like you feel . . ."
"It seems as if you . . ."
"You appear to be feeling . . ."
"I get the impression that . . ."

The feelings that the listener has perceived are used in each response. Lists of over 200 feeling words have been composed. This technique allows the listener to check the accuracy of his perceptions, and if they are wrong, the person will usually be quick to correct the perception. Usually no offense is taken and the person is happy that someone cared enough to try to understand.

BARRIERS TO EFFECTIVE COMMUNICATION

Patients can be frustrated by the inability to discuss their medication problems with the pharmacist. A common example is the patient who visits the doctor and receives a new prescription but forgets the instructions given. The patient then brings the prescription to the pharmacy with the idea of asking the pharmacist about the medication. However, the patient's weak attempt to communicate with the pharmacist is frustrated by a clerk. Often the role of the clerk is to receive the prescription from the patient, gather demographic information, and simply ask the patient, "Would you like counseling with that?" Other patients listening nearby may then non-verbally express a desire for an answer that will allow them to be waited on sooner. Meanwhile, the pharmacist (often in an elevated area behind a high counter, glass enclosed) is busy typing on the computer with one hand and holding the telephone with the other, completely ignoring or unaware of the activity at the counter. The patient receives the finished prescription without a word from the pharmacist or even from the clerk, who only collects payment. Thus, the patient goes home with a confused idea of how to use the medication.

This example illustrates how communication barriers impair effective communication in a community pharmacy. These barriers can be described as environmental (physical), psychological, administrative, or time conflict. Environmental barriers are basically physical in nature and will be discussed further in Chapter 5, "The Counseling Environment and Design."

PSYCHOLOGICAL BARRIERS

Psychological barriers include: semantics (different interpretations of the meanings of words), perception differences, inadequate feedback, and pharmacist attitudes.

Semantics

Semantics relate to the meanings of words and symbols used in interpersonal communication. Words only have meanings in terms of people's reactions to them. A particular word will mean different things to different patients depending on how it is used. There are two types of barriers associated with semantics. First, some words or phrases can have multiple interpretations, for example, the response of some patients to the use of the word "drug." Pharmacists use the term to refer to medications, while many patients associate the word with illicit or addictive compounds. Secondly, groups of health professionals develop their own technical language, not easily understood by lay persons. For example, pharmacists use acronyms like Rx, ADR, DUR, which only pharmacists may understand. Thus, because of frequent misinterpretations of this language, effective patient communication requires the use of words that are carefully chosen, while jargon should be clearly defined or avoided.

Perception Differences

How a message is viewed by a patient is called perception. Each individual's perception is unique and influenced by his or her own world. As a result, people may perceive a situation in entirely different ways. Variations in value systems also cause patients to respond to the same message in different ways. Thus, patients can be expected to react differently to messages because no two individuals have the same personal experiences, memories, fears, likes, and dislikes. If patients perceive a pharmacist to lack adequate drug or clinical knowledge, they are less likely either to ask questions or listen to advice offered. Alternatively, if the patient perceives the pharmacist as knowledgeable and has positive experiences, then the patient is more likely to seek the pharmacist's advice. Other potentially negative perceptions that a patient may have of a pharmacist include the following:

1. Pharmacists are only interested in diseases, drugs, and dollars, not people.
2. Patients may believe that everything they need to know from the pharmacist about their medications is typed on the prescription label.
3. The patient may consider their condition to be minor and to warrant no further discussion.
4. Patients may be so distraught from their condition that they are unable to talk with the pharmacist.

Feedback

The process in which information flows from the receiver back to the sender is called feedback. It helps the sender know if the receiver has received the correct message. For example, in order to learn if a patient has understood what he or she has been told, the pharmacist would ask the patient to explain in his or her own words what was heard. Just asking if he or she understands how to use the medication places the patient on the defensive and often results in little or no feedback. While the absence of feedback allows the pharmacist to deliver the counseling message more quickly, it does so at the cost of patient understanding. It may take longer, but it improves both the accuracy of and confidence in the message. Consequently, receipt and response to feedback, although more time consuming, can improve the quality of the communication.

Pharmacist Attitudes

A lack of confidence and low self-esteem can influence how pharmacists communicate. Pharmacists who do not believe they can communicate, or who did not know the right information to tell, or who are shy, or who have had bad communication experiences, tend to avoid communicating with patients. Pharmacists need to realize that communication is far from ideal all the time, and that they should strive to improve their communication skills through practice.

Fear of not being in control of a communication situation is another attitude barrier. This communication apprehension impairs a pharmacist's willingness to talk to patients for fear of making a mistake. Typically these fears are blown out of proportion in the pharmacist's mind, and when the situation is confronted, it usually turns out better than expected. The pharmacist's attitude towards dispensing versus counseling can also stymie good communication. Those who perceive dispensing to be more important than counseling will communicate less and eventually less effectively. Many pharmacists believe that talking with patients is not their job. Finally, many believe that patients neither expect nor want to be counseled.

ADMINISTRATIVE BARRIERS

Management may view the lack of direct financial compensation for communication activities as a powerful disincentive. Clearly, there are financial costs associated with patient counseling. If the pharmacist doesn't counsel, he or she can spend more time on tasks that generate income (e.g., fill more prescriptions). Thus, pharmacists are only supposed to dispense, since they are currently not compensated for counseling patients. Current dispensing processes make communication with patients difficult. Pharmacists complete a series of clerical and data entry tasks when dispensing that compete with the need to discuss the prescription with the patient. The removal of these administrative barriers may depend on the willingness of management and staff to alter work practices to facilitate the counseling task. This is much more likely to occur in today's community practice settings due to the compliance mandates of OBRA'90 concerning patient counseling.

TIME BARRIERS

Time constraints are interlinked with administrative barriers since management is responsible for staffing levels and the allocation of work duties. Both pharmacists and patients often have time conflicts and other time limitations. Thus, counseling at an inappropriate time is likely to fall short. For example, the pharmacist may have ten prescriptions waiting to be dispensed and a doctor wanting to give a prescription order by telephone, and a patient needs to be counseled. In another instance, a patient may have already waited for several hours in the doctor's office and is running late for work.

Yet, while time constraints are often used as an excuse not to counsel, counseling rarely lasts longer than two minutes per session. In addition, written information can be easily generated to supplement and reinforce a brief verbal message. Alternatively, the patient can be asked to return at a more convenient time or can be contacted by telephone.

The Counseling Environment and Design

Interactive patient medication counseling enhances information exchange and prompts effective learning by patients about their medications. But where it takes place is important. Before designing an effective patient counseling environment, it is necessary to identify the specific elements in the pharmacy that impede or facilitate good communication.

Lack of privacy is a good example of a significant barrier that impedes patient interaction and understanding. However, when designing a patient counseling area a separate room is not necessarily required. Actually, patients may be reluctant and uneasy about a separate, walled-off space. Nevertheless, there needs to be an effective consultation area, even one that is just adjacent to the prescription counter or separated from the merchandise area by a low wall or partition. Both pharmacist and patient can stand for most consultations, perhaps with the pharmacist standing just slightly elevated in front of the patient on a riser or platform. Chairs could be placed in a nearby area to allow patients to wait comfortably but out of hearing range.

ENVIRONMENTAL BARRIERS

Like privacy, the environment in which counseling takes place influences its process and outcome. Many environmental barriers are obvious such as those which are distracting, while others are more subtle. Physical barriers are the most common environmental barriers. Some environmental barriers that negatively affect patient counseling are listed in Table 5.1.

These barriers may have been originally designed to provide a safe work environment without interruption from waiting patients. Unfortunately, they also inhibit patients from gaining access to the pharmacist. These kinds

TABLE 5.1. Environmental Barriers Negatively Affecting Counseling.

1. Physical barriers between patients and pharmacists
a.   Counters in front of the dispensing counter
b.   Glass partitions separating the pharmacist from the patient
c.   A clerk or technician acting as a gatekeeper (positioned between the pharmacist and the patient)
2. Objects for pharmacists to hide behind
a.   Tall dispensing counters
b.   Computer screens
c.   Signs, printed material, or merchandise on counters obscuring view of the pharmacist
3. Problems making conversation difficult
a.   Noise from cash registers, telephones, computer printers or background music
b.   Distance between pharmacist and the patient requiring loud voices or yelling to hear
c.   Constant interruptions by staff or the telephone ringing
d.   A lack of privacy
e.   A sense of time urgency created by waiting patients and congestion around the dispensing area
4. Images discouraging communication
a.   Elevated dispensing areas
b.   Small windows for communications
c.   Pharmacist not easily identifiable (absence of a name badge or white coat)

of environmental barriers can send a strong message to patients that pharmacists are not interested in talking with them.

Often, environmental barriers must be identified before they can be removed. It has been suggested that the best way to do this is to put yourself in the place of the patient and ask yourself:

1. Can you actually see the pharmacist?
2. How difficult is it to get the pharmacist's attention?
3. Is the prescription area a place where you can converse in private?
4. Do you have to speak to a third person before you can talk to the pharmacist?
5. Are there too many distractions or too much noise?

These barriers can also increase the amount of effort required to effectively perform patient counseling. Thus, impeding physical barriers between patients and pharmacists must be removed, whenever possible without compromising security. For example, all objects used by pharmacists to hide behind should be removed from counters and dispensary benches. Patients need to be able to identify the pharmacist. Thus, pharmacists should wear name badges and white jackets to facilitate this.

Noise problems that may impair conversation are more difficult to deal with; however, it is usually possible to set aside a quiet corner or a partitioned area for patient consultation. Images that discourage effective communication should be removed wherever possible. For example, while highly elevated dispensing counters are useful for storage security, they create the perception that the pharmacist is always looking down at the patient. Patient medication consultation is always more effective when the pharmacist is both close to the patient and nearly at eye-level.

DESIGNING A PATIENT COUNSELING AREA

Once most environmental barriers are removed or reduced to a minimum, the prescription department can be considered ready to counsel patients. This is what designing a pharmacy for patient counseling basically accomplishes. There are several design factors that should always be employed for an effective counseling area. The height of the counter facing the patient should allow the patient to talk with the pharmacists at nearly eye-level. A height of fifty-four to sixty inches may be satisfactory. The computer or computer terminal must be placed next to, or be part of, the counseling area. Sufficient space should be provided to accommodate the important computer hardware. This is necessary for easy access to the patient's medication profile. Also, the pharmacist must be able to use the computer without having to bend over.

Most importantly, the counseling area must be located adjacent to the dispensing counter. This allows the pharmacist to move freely and easily from prescription-filling duties to patient counseling. The counseling area should be at the end of the dispensing counter to assure privacy. It should be delineated by a low wall to further assure privacy, but should be easily identified by the patient. A waiting area, with comfortable chairs and useful reading materials, can be nearby. However, those waiting should not be able to overhear or observe a counseling session. Ancillary pamphlets or literature for use in medication counseling can also be present nearby.

While it is probably unnecessary, the services of a pharmacy design consultant might be useful. They are available through fixture suppliers. An effective patient medication counseling area will help to provide optimal and efficient patient counseling and help the pharmacist comply with federal and counseling requirements. But perhaps best of all, it will produce more satisfied customers who are more likely to remain loyal to the pharmacy, which in turn may result in increased prescription volume.

CHAPTER 6

The Use of Pharmacy Technicians in Patient Counseling

PHARMACY TECHNICIAN TASKS

A major rationale for using pharmacy technicians in community pharmacy practice is to relieve the pharmacist of routine, non-judgmental, and non-discretionary tasks so that the pharmacist may counsel patients and perform other prescriptive and professional duties. Pharmacy technicians are generically referred to as ``supportive personnel,`` ``pharmacy support staff,`` or by some similar designation. They are employees of the pharmacy who have been trained on the job to assist the pharmacist, under the pharmacist's supervision, in the prescription department.

The supervised tasks that technicians are permitted to do will vary, depending on individual state statute or regulation. However, the following are a cross section of these permitted duties:

1. Retrieval of prescriptions or files as needed (may include counting and pouring under supervision)
2. Clerical tasks such as typing labels and maintaining patient profiles (may allow affixing the label to the prescription container)
3. Secretarial tasks such as telephoning, filing and typing
4. Accounting tasks such as recordkeeping, maintaining accounts receivables, third-party reimbursements and posting
5. Inventory control tasks including monitoring, pricing, dating, invoicing, stocking pharmacy and preparation of purchase orders
6. Maintenance of a clean and orderly pharmacy
7. Requesting, receiving and recording prescription refill information
8. Initiation of counseling requests or refusals

At least forty-one states currently allow technicians to enter information into patient profiles, which are usually checked by a pharmacist. The pharmacist remains responsible for the completeness and accuracy of the entry. State regulations also prohibit pharmacy technicians from performing specific duties that are normally reserved for the pharmacist. Duties prohibited to a technician include the following. A technician:

1. Cannot interpret the prescription
2. Cannot do any compounding or reconstitution
3. Cannot prepare any intravenous, enteral or other sterile medications
4. Cannot order, stock, dispense or perform any other physical tasks involving Schedule II controlled substances
5. Cannot counsel patients

PHARMACY TECHNICIAN TRAINING PROGRAMS

State boards of pharmacy are requiring pharmacies to develop and conduct training programs for their pharmacy technicians. The participating pharmacies are required to attest to a technician's successful completion of a program.

A typical attestation form for indicating successful completion of a pharmacy technician training program is one adapted from the pharmacy technician program of the Louisiana State Board of Pharmacy (see Figure 6.1).

Guidelines for the development of pharmacy technician training programs also have been established by many state boards of pharmacy. These guidelines might be summarized to reflect the following training categories:

1. Orientation to pharmacy practice
2. Duties of pharmacy personnel
3. Communication techniques
4. Understanding state pharmacy laws, rules and regulations
5. Pharmaceutical, mathematical and drug terminology
6. Pharmaceutics for pharmacy technicians
7. Basic pharmacology
8. Handling medications
9. Basics of medication dispensing
10. Repackaging and manufacturing functions
11. Financial and claims activities

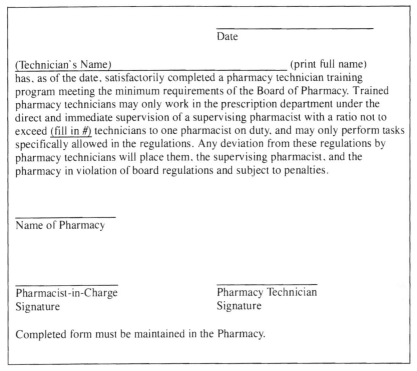

Date

(Technician's Name) _____ (print full name)
has, as of the date, satisfactorily completed a pharmacy technician training
program meeting the minimum requirements of the Board of Pharmacy. Trained
pharmacy technicians may only work in the prescription department under the
direct and immediate supervision of a supervising pharmacist with a ratio not to
exceed <u>(fill in #)</u> technicians to one pharmacist on duty, and may only perform tasks
specifically allowed in the regulations. Any deviation from these regulations by
pharmacy technicians will place them, the supervising pharmacist, and the
pharmacy in violation of board regulations and subject to penalties.

Name of Pharmacy

Pharmacist-in-Charge   Pharmacy Technician
Signature   Signature

Completed form must be maintained in the Pharmacy.

FIGURE 6.1. Pharmacy technician training program statement of completeness and understanding

PHARMACIST LIABILITY

Most state regulations limit the number of pharmacy technicians that can
be on duty at any time. This is usually expressed as a ratio of technicians
per registered pharmacist. Several states permit a 3 to 1 ratio of technicians
per pharmacist. However, in most states the ratio is one technician for each
pharmacist on duty. Violation of these ratios or any violation committed by
a pharmacy technician may subject the supervising pharmacist to penalties.
These penalties may include license and/or permit revocation or suspension.

The supervising pharmacist also may be legally responsible for the acts
of the supervised technician under the legal concept of *respondent superior*.
This is most likely to apply if it can be proven that the pharmacist is
exercising control over the conduct of the pharmacy technician. The extent
to which this may actually happen may be directly related to the amount of
prescriptive and counseling duties that technicians are allowed to perform
in the pharmacy. Basically, what this means is that any unsupervised tech-

nician act that may result in an injury to a patient may cause legal action to be instituted against the supervising pharmacist. Sanctions that could apply include malpractice suits and possible criminal prosecution.

NEW INCENTIVES FOR USING PHARMACY TECHNICIANS

OBRA'90 mandates are also affecting the use of pharmacy technicians in the community pharmacy. Rapidly increasing involvement of pharmacists in patient counseling and prospective drug utilization review activities is already motivating state boards of pharmacy to permit technicians to perform expanded prescriptive duties. Eventually, this may result in that which has already occurred in other areas, such as radiology and pathology, where technicians perform basic functional, professional duties. Thus, in the future, pharmacy technicians may be filling prescriptions, while pharmacists are counseling patients.

Recent interpretations of OBRA'90 mandates also suggest that pharmacy technicians will be allowed to participate in patient counseling activities. The Health Care Financing Administration (HCFA) has stated that pharmacy technicians may be allowed to initiate patient counseling requests for pharmacists or obtain patient refusals for counseling. While actual counseling of patients may be prohibited, technician involvement will free the pharmacist's time, greatly enhancing the ability of the pharmacist to successfully counsel.

CHAPTER 7

Patient Medication Profile Development

It is likely that today's patient is taking medications prescribed by more than one physician. Often these physicians will not be aware that their patients are receiving medications prescribed by other doctors. With a greater number taking medications, there is also a greater probability of patients having drug interactions, allergies, idiosyncrasies, and adverse reactions. Thus, it has become necessary for the pharmacist to have full knowledge of all the medications a patient may be taking. Of course, it would be helpful if the patient could have all of his or her prescriptions filled by a single pharmacy. Yet a patient's medication therapy also may be monitored effectively by keeping a record of the patient's medication history and other pertinent patient information. Indeed, patient profiles may have become a necessary part of many community pharmacy practices.

There are several reasons for having a patient profile system in your pharmacy. Of course, many states legally require their pharmacies to maintain patient profiles. These are mandatory patient profile systems. However, many pharmacies in states not mandating profiles still utilize them. Among other important reasons for using a profile is the need to document a patient's medication history in order to monitor and promote medication compliance. It also acts as a data source, providing information that can be utilized by health-care professionals to solve medication use problems for the general public.

THE NATURE OF PATIENT PROFILE SYSTEMS

The type and amount of information found in a patient medication profile will vary among pharmacies. It often depends upon the nature of individual pharmacist-patient relationships. The literature suggests that there may be ten informational elements present in the typical patient profile:

1. History of adverse effects
2. Potentially unwarranted/unintended changes in therapeutic regimen
3. Potential quantitative misuse (non-compliance, misuse, overuse)
4. Duplication of medications
5. Additive effects from similar medication use
6. Inappropriate dosage, route of administration, dosing schedule or dosage form
7. Potential current adverse effects
8. Drug-drug interactions
9. Drug-disease interactions
10. Irrational therapeutic regimen

In addition, the basic categories of information that should be available on the patient profile probably include:

- *Patient Demographics*
  Name, address, phone number, birthdate/age
- *Clinical Problems/Conditions*
  Drug allergies, idiosyncrasies, side effects, disease/condition
- *Practitioner Demographics*
  Name and specialty of prescriber, pharmacist identification, etc.
- *Medication Information*
  Previous medication therapy, current medication therapy (product name, dosage form, strength and quantity dispensed, etc.)
- *Financial Information*
  Medication charges, tax information, insurance transactions

CONSIDERATIONS IN THE EFFECTIVE USE OF THE PROFILE

1. *Type of Profile* – The pharmacist must choose which profile system most likely fits his or her practice needs. Two basic types are the family and the individual profiles. The family system allows all household members to be listed on a single file. The individual profile alleviates patient monitoring and is less subject to mistakes and confusion. There is also the question of whether to use a manual or a computer-based profile system. However, with the need to handle large amounts of patient information in today's practice settings, computer systems are more apt to assure that the patient profile is current and accessible.

2. *Confidentiality* – The confidentiality of the medication profile should be maintained on a par with that of the filled prescription. Information originating from the profile can be given in good faith, but only when the pharmacist feels that it is in the best interest of the patient. Manual profile systems are able to handle problems of confidentiality by separating potentially sensitive information (e.g., patient condition) from the non-sensitive (tax or insurance information). Computer systems can be easily programmed for confidentiality protection.

3. *Using the Profile as a Management Tool* – The patient medication profile also can be used to generate information for use in effective pharmacy management. Third-party payment data, preparation of tax and insurance records, billing information, etc. may provide useful information to assist in inventory control, purchasing decisions, or in the determination of medication costs and prices. In essence, good business practices can use the information provided by a good patient profile system.

LEGAL CONSIDERATIONS

A majority of states still do not mandate their pharmacies to maintain patient profiles (but see ``Effects of OBRA'90 on Patient Medication Profiles''). Table 7.1 lists the nineteen states that currently do require patient profiles.

While keeping a patient profile might expose the pharmacist to additional liability, it is equally possible that failure to do so would subject the pharmacist to further liability. It could be argued that the pharmacist's knowledge and expertise in medication management (e.g., detection of drug-drug interactions) already obligates him or her to use profile information without actually maintaining one. The maintenance of some kind of profile system may have become today's accepted standard of pharmacy practice. Thus, a pharmacist who dispenses a prescription and makes no attempt to record a potential drug-drug interaction may be exposing himself to a malpractice suit, if the patient suffers a serious reaction to the medication.

The issue of confidentiality reflects the legal right of a person to privacy. Pharmacists have an obligation not to reveal patient profile information without the patient's consent. Generally, only the patient's physician or officers of the law have legal permission to obtain that kind of information. Privacy among family members must be considered. This also applies to minors who, when legally permitted, may prohibit divulgence of informa-

TABLE 7.1. States That Mandate Patient Medication Profiles.

Arkansas	
California	
Delaware	Use profile for each prescription
Idaho	Or a daily patient log
Iowa	
Kansas	Only for pharmacies in adult-care facility
Maine	Use profile for each prescription
Minnesota	
New Jersey	Use profile for each prescription
New York	
North Dakota	Use profile for each prescription
Oregon	
Tennessee	
Utah	
Vermont	
Washington	
Wisconsin	May use to keep refill records
(Florida)	Pending
(Nebraska)	Pending

tion to their parents, and to spouses who may become involved in divorce or custody situations.

EFFECTS OF OBRA'90 UPON PATIENT MEDICATION PROFILES

There is little doubt that the OBRA`90 regulations mandate the use of some kind of patient medication record under prospective drug utilization review (ProDUR). At least the following applies to all patients whose prescriptions are filled under Medicaid:

> The pharmacist must also make a reasonable effort to obtain and record patient information and maintain the patient profiles that are essential for the pharmacist to counsel the recipient concerning medication problems unique to the recipient.

This need for a profile system stems from the OBRA`90 requirement to review a patient's drug therapy before each Medicaid prescription is filled. This review includes screening for potential drug problems due to:

- therapeutic duplication
- drug-disease contraindication
- adverse drug-drug interaction
- incorrect drug dosage
- incorrect duration of drug treatment
- drug-allergy interactions
- clinical abuse/misuse

Based upon these considerations, ``A pharmacist conducting ProDUR can use the patient profile to obtain information from the patient about allergies, disease conditions, and other relevant information.'' In addition, it is reasonable to expect pharmacists, who follow ProDUR procedures and counsel *all* patients, to utilize patient profiles.

The recordkeeping requirements of the Act specify that each state ``must require that, in case of Medicaid recipients, the pharmacist make a reasonable effort to obtain, record, and maintain patient profiles'' containing at least the following:

- Name, address, telephone number, date of birth (or age), and gender of the patient
- Individual medical history, if significant, including disease state or states, known allergies and drug reactions, and a comprehensive list of medications and relevant devices
- Pharmacist's comments relevant to the individual's drug therapy

This type of documentation could be useful for non-Medicaid patients as well. The OBRA'90 regulations do recognize limitations in obtaining the above ``individual medical history,'' noting that the pharmacist does not have ``direct access to diagnosis information and details about disease conditions contained in medical records available in an inpatient environment.'' Nevertheless, the pharmacist is expected to access sufficient information to fulfill review and screening obligations. A patient medication profile can provide the needed tool to do this.

A MODEL FOR PATIENT MEDICATION PROFILES

Currently, the mandates of OBRA'90 remain the major impetus behind the growing utilization of patient profiles. Nevertheless, there are any number of good reasons to use a single, practical profile record system to accommodate professional, economic, and legal needs. The model for such a system is probably the one developed by the National Association of Boards of Pharmacy (N.A.B.P.). It essentially fulfills all legal and OBRA'90

TABLE 7.2. A Model for a Patient Record of Medications Profile (PROMP).

A. Introduction
    1. The patient record of medications profile (PROMP) allows for immediate and easy retrieval of information necessary to the dispensing pharmacist for identifying medications previously dispensed, and for counseling purposes before the current prescription order is dispensed.

B. Patient and Medications Identification
    1. The following patient information should be available for medication identification and counseling:
        a. Full name of the patient for whom the medication is intended
        b. Address and telephone number of the patient
        c. Patient's age or date of birth
        d. Patient's gender
        e. A list of prescriptions dispensed previously to the patient during the five years immediately preceding the most recent entry. The list should show the following:
            (1) Name of the medication
            (2) Prescription number
            (3) Name and strength of the medication
            (4) The quantity and date dispensed
            (5) The name and specialty of the prescriber
            (6) The indication(s) for use
        f. A record of the pharmacist's comments relevant to the patient's medication therapy including any information relevant to the patient or to any medication currently being dispensed, such as:
            (1) Caregiver identification
            (2) Counseling documentation
            (3) Refill instruction and/or history
            (4) Missed doses history
            (5) Record of counseling offers
            (6) Pharmacist-prescriber interaction

C. Prospective Drug Review (ProDUR) Information
    1. The pharmacist shall record information pertaining to the patient's medical history obtained from the patient or the patient's caregiver for use in Prospective Drug Review (ProDUR) including the following:
        a. Allergies
        b. Adverse drug reactions (common, serious side effects)
        c. Idiosyncrasies
        d. Chronic conditions
        e. Disease states
        f. Currently used prescription medications
        g. Currently used over-the-counter medications (OTCs)
        h. Currently used medical devices

TABLE 7.2. (continued).

D. Documentation Requirements
1. The Patient Record of Medications Profile shall be maintained for a period of not less than *five years* from the date of the last entry in the profile record (or your state requirements)
2. This record may be a hard copy or a computerized form.
3. Reasons for not counseling must be recorded. This includes refusal due to prescriber request or in response to the patient/caregiver.
E. Administrative and Financial Information
1. Tax records
2. Insurance records
3. Billing information
F. Miscellaneous
(individualized for *your* pharmacy)

requirements, and the professional needs of pharmacists who are motivated to practice pharmaceutical care in their communities. It is interesting to note that many of the states which currently mandate patient profiles, and those responding to the mandates of OBRA'90, have developed their profile requirements to reflect that of the N.A.B.P. model. We believe that this model or one like it should be adopted by all pharmacies and modified to suit their own practice needs. Accordingly, we have modified it to one that we feel is well suited for use by pharmacists in *counseling patients*. We call it the "Patient Record of Medications Profile" or PROMP (Table 7.2).

CHAPTER 8

The Prescription Label

THE PRESCRIPTION ORDER

It would be very unfortunate if the most carefully conceived and constructed prescription becomes therapeutically useless because it was miscommunicated to the patient and not followed as intended. Prescriber and pharmacist each has a responsibility to properly and completely inform patients about their drug therapy. Thus, effective and consistent communication between the physician and the pharmacist, on behalf of the patient, is desirable.

The prescription order is the vehicle through which the medication needs of the patient are most effectively and consistently communicated from prescriber to the pharmacist. The pharmacist uses the prescription to precisely fill the order and to provide the necessary information and assistance to ensure patient compliance. It also provides the means for the pharmacist to advise the prescriber of any problems associated with the nature of the order or potentially undesirable effects on the patient.

COMPONENTS OF THE PRESCRIPTION ORDER

The prescription is generally defined as a medication order issued by a duly, state-licensed practitioner such as a physician, dentist, or veterinarian. This order is usually intended for a specific individual, in a specific amount or form, to be used in a specific manner, for a specified amount of time, and for a specific purpose or indication. It represents that medical decision which both patient and prescriber believe will result in maximizing desired therapeutic outcomes, i.e., curing disease, alleviating pain, relieving stress, and improving the quality of life.

The prescription components are easy to identify and follow a pattern and order that remain essentially the same for any prescription. This pattern should allow for easy interpretation to maximize the accuracy of the information being transmitted from the prescriber to the pharmacist. Traditionally, prescriptions are written on a printed form, or prescription blank, which facilitates the ordering of these components. Some components may be preprinted on the blank with prescriber-specific information such as name, address and DEA number. The remaining components are written in other specific sections of the blank when prescribed. Thus, all components are usually found in the same parts of the prescription each and every time a prescription is written.

The parts of the prescription are as follows:

1. Prescriber information
2. Patient information
3. Date of issue
4. The Rx symbol (the superscription)
5. Medication that is prescribed (the inscription)
6. Dispensing directions to pharmacist (the subscription)
7. Directions for the patients (the signatura, signa, or sig.)
8. Labeling and other directions
9. Refill information
10. Prescriber's signature

Prescriber Information

This information usually includes the prescriber's name or office title, address, telephone number, degree(s), and DEA number for prescriptions of controlled substances. It may be preprinted and is found on the top of the prescription blank. However, the DEA number and prescriber's name are commonly found at the bottom, immediately following the space for the physician's signature.

Patient Information

Proper patient identification is, of course, necessary to avoid any confusion with medications intended for specific persons. The patient's age may be useful for assuring the dispensing of appropriate dosages and dosage forms. Prescriptions for controlled substances require the patient's name and address to be correctly identified. This information is often omitted by prescribers and routinely added by pharmacists.

Date of Issue

Written prescriptions are normally dated when they are issued by the prescriber to the patient. This establishes a specific time-frame that assists the pharmacist in determining the continued medication needs of the patient. It also helps the pharmacist to adhere to the six months or five refills limitation for controlled substances and time limitations in other instances.

The Rx Symbol (Superscription) and Prescribed Medication (Inscription)

The Rx symbol or superscription generally precedes the inscription, or the name, dosage form and strength of the prescribed medication. This may be appropriately referred to as the body of the prescription order. The Rx symbol, of course, is the universally recognized notation for identifying ``a prescription'' and other pharmaceutical designations. This symbol is thought to be a contraction of the Latin verb, *recipe*. Unless compounding is required, most inscriptions are for already prepared dosage forms. These medications are most often prescribed by their brand names. However, the evolution of drug product selection and other incentives have encouraged the growing use of generic names and products.

Dispensing Directions (Subscription)

This component is particularly important when compounding requires prescribers to communicate explicit directions to the pharmacist on the ingredients to be mixed, the dosage form to be made, and the amounts to be dispensed. The use of prepared pharmaceuticals have all but reduced this component to identifying the number of dosage units to be dispensed. Nevertheless, this number can be useful as an indicator of length of medication therapy.

Patient Directions (Signatura)

The prescriber provides the patient with the directions for correctly using the medication in this portion of the prescription order called the signatura (sig.). These directions are usually written using abbreviated English and/or Latin words. Here are some examples:

- Caps ii q 4 h (*Take 2 capsules every four hours.*)
- gtts. iii ou pc & hs (*Place 3 drops in both eyes after meals and at bedtime.*)
- Apply sparingly QID (*Apply sparingly to affected area four times a day.*)

As can be seen by the interpretations (given parenthetically in *italics*), the pharmacist's job is to transform these terms into readily understood and easily followed instructions. In addition, these interpretations must be consistent with what the patient may remember from the visit with the prescriber. This may not always be as simple a task as it may seem (see p. 50). Nevertheless, prescriber guidelines suggest that the following considerations should always be addressed in the directions:

1. Write in English; Latin serves no useful purpose.
2. Use commonly understood abbreviations.
3. Avoid ''as directed'' and similar expressions.
4. Indicate specific times of the day for taking medications.
5. Associate patient needs with age, handicaps, and language difficulties.

Label and Refill Instructions

This is important information especially for pharmacists in those states requiring that the name, strength, and quantity of the medication dispensed be placed on the prescription label. Hopefully, the advantages of this rapid identification of the medication will encourage prescribers to permit its use and allow pharmacists to include this information routinely on the label. Some prescription blanks are imprinted with the word ''label,'' followed by a space for prescribers to indicate their permission. In addition, information such as expiration date, lot number, or storage instructions may be required on the label in the future.

Only the prescriber can authorize refills. Specific refill instructions are necessary so that the pharmacist can legally and professionally decide the extent to which prescription orders are refillable. The five refills or six-month limitation on controlled substances should be followed. Federal law and many states do not recognize the use of such designations as ''PRN,'' which may tempt a pharmacist to authorize inappropriate or illegal refills. Fortunately, state law often informs the pharmacist on how to handle such problems by defining a maximum refill period for prescriptions (e.g., one year).

Prescriber Signature and Additional Information

Ordinarily, the prescriber's signature is necessary for completing the prescription order. Others (nurses, pharmacists, office personnel) may sign the prescription for the physician; however, prescriptions for Schedule II controlled substances require the prescriber's original signature. Nevertheless, the authorization to prescribe all original orders or refills remains with the prescriber. A pharmacist may be held legally responsible for not recognizing this.

THE PRESCRIPTION LABEL

The prescription label is the fundamental means for communicating important information to patients about their medications. The best label leaves the least interpretation to the patient. Thus, the pharmacist always must provide a clear and concise label, and one that the patient will readily understand.

Prescriber guidelines recommend that the following information be placed on the prescription label:

1. Name and strength of the medication prescribed
2. Specific times a day for administration
3. Specific dosage intervals when appropriate
4. Appropriate route of administration
5. Symptom, indication, or intended effect for which the medication is prescribed
6. Precise refill information (avoid PRN)
7. Complete patient information
8. Carefully worded directions for use (no confusing abbreviations or vague instructions, e.g. "as directed")

In response to these guidelines, pharmacists have traditionally placed the following information on prescription labels:

1. Pharmacy name, address and telephone number
2. Name of prescriber (include specialty identification when possible)
3. Name and strength of medication dispensed (use name most familiar to patient)
4. Directions for use
5. Prescription number
6. Date dispensed
7. Patient's name

8. Refill information (e.g., number remaining, approximate date of next refill)

In addition, the following information might be required or appropriate for the prescription label:

1. Intended route of administration
2. Expiration date or lot number
3. Special storage information
4. Special cautions or warnings
5. Pharmacist's name

DIRECTIONS-FOR-USE

All label information is important. However, the directions-for-use may be the most important component of the label. The doctor uses the label instructions to tell the patient what to do with the medication and how to use it correctly. There are no specific legal requirements for what actually must be included in any labeled direction-for-use, except what is vaguely stated as, ''the directions for use contained in the prescription.'' *It is up to the prescriber to decide what is to be included.* This literally forces the pharmacist to be very careful in interpreting what the doctor is trying to tell the patient. Thus, there is a compelling need on the part of the pharmacist to be able to identify specific parts of the directions-for-use in order to simplify this task. Legal and professional sources suggest that the following easily recognized components be used routinely for prescription label directions-for-use:

1. Quantity of dose and dosage form
2. Route of administration
3. Time of administration
4. Frequency of administration
5. Duration of administration
6. Intended use
7. Preparation for use

Effect of the Prescription Directions-for-Use on Patient Compliance

The directions for taking the medication may have an important impact on patient compliance. Yet the best motivated patients cannot be compliant by following directions they cannot read, do not understand, or find incomplete and jumbled. It appears improbable that a conscientious patient would spend a considerable amount of money to get help from a physician and not follow the doctor's instructions to take medication correctly. Thus, while it does happen, it is unfair to suggest that the patient alone is at fault for failing to comply.

Perhaps patients do understand how their medications are to be used, at the time of the doctor's visit. Frequently, when asked, patients will say that they understood how to take their medications, or that the doctor told them how to medicate themselves. Yet the average patient forgets half of the prescriber's instructions by the time he or she gets to the pharmacy. Even when leaving the pharmacy, patients may be still unclear about the doctor's instructions, or have forgotten vital information on how to take costly medications, *unless* there are specific directions to do so on the prescription label. The words chosen for the label instructions must reflect precisely what the physician intended for the patient as well. Indeed, patients expect their pharmacists to help them recall and follow the physician's instructions.

The pharmacist should not assume that the patient or caregiver adequately understands how to correctly use a medication without a proper label to serve as a constant reminder. At the same time, that label gives the pharmacist the opportunity to provide the patient with other useful information about the medication, such as proper usage of dosage forms (removing the suppository wrapping, shake well instruction, using inhalers and patches, etc.). Remember, the patient's understanding of the treatment is as important as an understanding of the disease itself.

ABBREVIATIONS AND PUNCTUATION USE

Prescriber and pharmacist guidelines officially discourage the use of confusing abbreviations. Actually, there is no "official" list of abbreviations for use on the prescription label. Yet prescribers and pharmacists routinely use them. Many are derived from Latin and English, while others may be shorthand creations of individual prescribers. A pharmacist should *never* guess at the potentially unrecognizable meanings of abbreviations.

Prescribers use common abbreviations for medication names, diseases, conditions, and for a variety of other things (e.g. "BM" for bowel movement, "ATC" for around-the-clock) in prescription writing. Abbreviations commonly used in writing or labeling directions-for-use may be categorized into six types: time-related, anatomical, dosage form and administration, dose and strength, number, and miscellaneous (see Table 8.1.).

While they should be discouraged for use in prescription label directions, the following are important considerations when abbreviations may be used appropriately:

TABLE 8.1. Common Types of Prescription Label Abbreviations.

Time-related		Dose and Strength	
a.c.	– before meals	c.c.	– cubic centimeter
a.m.	– morning	gr.	– grain
h.	– hour	g.	– gram
h.s.	– at bedtime	gtt.	– drop
p.c.	– after meals	mcg.	– microgram
p.m.	– evening	mg.	– milligram
p.r.n.	– as needed	mL.	– milliliter
q.d.	– every day	tsp.	– one teaspoon
q.o.d.	– every other day	tbsp.	– one tablespoon
Anatomical		**Number**	
a.s.	– left ear	i-x	– one to ten
a.u.	– both ears	ss	– 1/2
o.s.	– left eye	L	– 50
o.u.	– both eyes	C	– 100
sl.	– under the tongue	M	– 1000
Dosage Form and Administration		**Miscellaneous**	
cap.	– capsule	a.a.	– of each
im.	– intramuscular	c.	– with
iv.	– intravenous	n.r.	– no refill
p.o.	– by mouth	q.s.	– sufficient quantity
sol.	– solution	s.	– without
sub-q.	– subcutaneously	stat	– immediately
supp.	– suppository	ut dict.	– as directed
syr.	– syrup		
tab.	– tablet		
ung.	– ointment		

1. Use generally accepted abbreviations, well understood by patients.
2. Use abbreviations only if necessary to shorten the directions.
3. A number preceding an abbreviation is separated by one space (25 mg.).
4. Ordinal numbers are not separated by a space (3rd, 10th).
5. Do not use abbreviations that may be used for two or more different words (min. for minim or minute).
6. Dose directions may use abbreviations for strength but not for dosage form (25 mg. is OK, but not one tab.).

7. The correct way to punctuate abbreviated words is to place the period after each word (im. not i.m., p.m. not pm.).

USING WORDS AND NAMES CORRECTLY

Names of medications and names of persons should always be capitalized. When using the name of a medication it is best to use the brand name or a name most familiar to the patient. The name should be as specific as possible. Thus, the medication name can be modified by adding descriptors to clarify it for the patient.

Darvocet-N® tablet
or
red Darvocet-N® tablet
or
Darvocet-N® (red tablet)

Furthermore, the actual medication name should be used only if the patient can recognize it. Otherwise specific descriptors well understood by the patient (i.e., little white tablet, long red tablet, etc.) are to be used. It is best to stay away from difficult words, vaguely understood words, and medical or pharmaceutical jargon. While some may be familiar with the medical terminology used by clinicians, equivalent lay terms would probably suit more patients. Table 8.2 lists difficult words and translations for use on prescription labels.

THE ORDERING OF LABEL INSTRUCTIONS

While the utility of clear, concise, and readily understandable instructions to insure patient medication compliance is widely recognized, low compliance rates continue to be reported. Perhaps misinterpretation of prescription label directions-for-use is due to inconsistency. If so, then presentation of these directions in an *orderly* fashion may help to resolve this matter. Simply put, the use of consistent ordering of the components of any directions-for-use should enhance comprehension. Like the pattern and order of the prescription itself, which maximizes the accuracy of the information being transmitted from the prescriber to the pharmacist, ordered prescription directions-for-use will maximize prescriber-to-pharmacist-to-patient communication.

There is also good reason to believe that patients *perceive and remember* information given to them in some kind of ordered fashion. There may be a mental pattern each patient has for best learning and remembering prescription instructions. Thus, directions for use of medications will be better understood and used when both patterns are merged.

TABLE 8.2. Difficult Word Categories.

Medical Jargon	Translation	Anatomical Words	Translation
Abrasions	Cuts, scrapes	Abdominal	Stomach
Agitation	Nervousness	Bowel	Gut
Angina	Chest pain	Buttocks	Buns, bottom
Anxiety	Nerves	Cardiac	Heart
Arrhythmia	Irregular heartbeat	Coccyx	Tail bone
Arthritis	Joint pain	Decubitus	Bed sore
Bradycardia	Slow heartbeat	Dorsal	Backside
Colic	Gas pains	Hemorrhoids	Piles
Congestion	Stuffy	Lesions	Sores
Diabetes	High blood sugar	Optic	Pertaining to eyes
Diarrhea	Loose stools, the "runs"	Otic	Pertaining to ears
Edema	Swelling	Navel	Belly button
Expectorate	Spit out	Penis	Private part (male)
Fever blisters	Cold sores	Prostate	"Nature"
Flatulence	Gas	Renal	Kidney
Glaucoma	Eye pressure	Thigh	Upper leg
Gout	Sore toe	Tumor	Growth
Hoarseness	Raspy voice	Urine	Pee
Hypertension	High blood pressure	Vagina	Private part (female)
Hypotension	Low blood pressure		
Instill	Put, place	**Vaguely**	
Indigestion	Upset stomach	**Understood**	**Translation**
Inflammation	Redness	Bedside	Next to bed
Inhale	Breath in	Bedtime	Just before sleep
Insomnia	Hard to sleep	Daily	Same time every day
Menstrual	Period	Dizziness	Spinning in head
Nausea	Stomach	Drowsiness	Sleepy
Nebulize	Spray	Fatal	Causing death
Palpitations	Rapid heartbeat	Inhibit	Slow down
Pre-menstrual	PMS	Itchy	Scratchy
Sinus	Nose cavity	Onset	Start of
Sublingually	Under the tongue	Persistent	Doesn't stop
Spasm	Cramp	Sparingly	A small amount
Subcutaneously	Under the skin		
Swish	Rinse		
Syncope	Fainting		
Tachycardia	Fast heartbeat		
Tension	Stress		
Tinnitus	Ringing in ears		
Vial	Pill bottle		
Vertigo	Head spinning		
Vomiting	Throwing up		

A. Oral Solids
   1. Take one capsule by mouth once daily at 8 a.m., until told to stop, for high blood pressure.
   2. Take one tablet by mouth 2 times a day at 8 a.m. and 8 p.m. for 8 weeks for ulcer.
B. Oral Liquids
   1. Take 1/2 teaspoon by mouth three times a day at 8 a.m., 2 p.m., and 10 p.m. for 7 days for infection.
   2. Take 2 tablespoons of the solution by mouth once a day at bedtime (11 p.m.) as needed for constipation.
C. Eye, Ear, and Nasal Solutions
   1. Place 2 drops in each eye 2 times a day at 8 a.m. and 8 p.m. every day for eye pressure.
   2. Place 2 drops in left ear 4 times a day at 7 a.m., 12 noon, 5 p.m., and 10 p.m., until gone, for infection.
   3. Put 3 drops into left nostril 2 times a day at 8 a.m. and 8 p.m. as needed for stuffy nose.
D. External Use Preparations
   1. Apply generously to warts 2 times a day at 8 a.m. and 8 p.m. to remove warts.
   2. Rub required amount into face 2 times a day in the morning and evening (8 a.m. and 8 p.m.) as needed to treat acne.
   3. Mix one teaspoonful in a pint of warm water and douche your private part every night at bedtime for up to 5 days.
   4. Use enough powder to dust the affected area 4 times a day at 7 a.m., 12 noon, 5 p.m. and 10 p.m. until infection is gone.
E. Miscellaneous
   1. Apply one patch to chest (different area each time) once a day at 8 a.m as needed for chest pain.
   2. Inject 15 units under the skin daily just before breakfast, until told to stop, for high blood sugar.
   3. Breath in 2 puffs by mouth 3 times a day at 8 a.m., 2 p.m., and 10 p.m. every day for asthma.

FIGURE 8.1   Ordered directions for use by dosage form

Analysis of prescription signatura ("sigs") suggests that an orderly system (or schema) for communicating label directions to the patient might take the following form:

1. Command verb (take, give, apply) (*You* is the understood subject.)
2. Amount and dosage form (one tablet, one suppository)
3. Method or route of administration (by mouth, under the tongue)
4. Frequency, duration, and time of administration (twice a day at 8 a.m., and 8 p.m. for ten days)

5. Indication for use (for cough, for relieving pain)
6. Addendum: usually a prepositional phrase expanding on one or more of the previous components (if pain persists after ten doses, stop)

An appropriate example of orderly label directions would be: "Take one tablet by mouth twice a day at 8 a.m. and 8 p.m. for ten days for ear infection, then call doctor."

All components should be included in the *same* order for the directions on any label. The specific wording would be determined by the prescriber, while the pharmacist would assure that the correct ordering appeared on the prescription label.

Ordered Directions-for-Use Samples

There will be differences in label directions-for-use among prescriptions. In addition to those of individual prescribers, these differences will depend mostly upon the nature of the medication prescribed, particularly, on the *dosage form*. However, there is no need to compromise the correct ordering of the directions-for-use when, for example, they are consistent with the proper use of the dosage form. In addition, when some directions-for-use allow for omission of one or more components, there is still no need to change the component order. To illustrate how to accommodate differences in label directions-for-use without compromising the correct order, refer to Figure 8.1.

CHAPTER 9

Counseling the Patient

The concept of pharmaceutical care and new national and state regulations are demanding radical changes in the everyday practice of pharmacy. Prospective drug utilization review requirements to counsel each and every patient will significantly change the work habits of pharmacists. Some pharmacists may respond that counseling is nothing new and that they have always provided it. However, closer examination reveals that this requirement changes the extent and liability of this service.

Until now the pharmacist chose which prescriptions and which patients to counsel. This service, once limited to a few, is now mandated for Medicaid patients and, by most states, for all patients. Most pharmacists can recall instances where they have assertively intervened in patient therapy and were satisfied with the results. The current regulations ask us to provide this level of service and intervention to each patient. Furthermore, these interventions, conversations, and analyses need to be documented. This new style of practice is consistent with the practice concept of pharmaceutical care. The new definition of pharmacy includes the existing definitions, the responsibility of getting the right drug to the right patient at the right time, and also expands the responsibilities of pharmacists to strive to achieve definite outcomes that will improve a patient's quality of life.

Patient counseling is just one task among new responsibilities for therapy outcomes. No longer is it acceptable to fill valid prescriptions for less than optimal therapy. Patient counseling is expected to improve medication compliance, avoid medication errors, improve outcomes of medication therapy, and reduce overall medication costs.

Patient counseling standards require major changes from past practices. The pharmacist must offer to discuss with each individual patient "whatever practical matters are deemed important," concerning medication needs. These important practical matters include:

- name and description of medication
- dosage form, route, and duration of therapy
- special directions and precautions
- side effects, adverse reactions, interactions and contraindications
- self-monitoring therapy
- proper storage
- refill information
- what to do for a missed dose

INTERACTIVE PATIENT MEDICATION COUNSELING

This book utilizes an interactive counseling system as the most practical and effective means of showing pharmacists how they can provide realistic patient medication counseling. The basis of any such system is the establishment of key informational areas. These areas should reflect subject matter that is routinely addressed in any patient counseling session. Traditionally, individual health-care providers have decided what is the nature of that subject matter. However, now it is being determined mostly through the patient counseling mandates of federal and state law.

The initial moments of an interactive patient counseling session often are the most awkward. The patient may be unaccustomed to discussing their health or medication needs with a pharmacist and may be hesitant or resistant at first. The pharmacist may have similar inclinations. The pharmacist needs to start the process by introducing himself or herself, and determining if the person who is receiving the prescription is the patient or caregiver. Then, the purpose of the counseling session should be stated. It is also reassuring to note the length of time needed to counsel. Hearing that it will take only two or three minutes may ease patient resistance and pharmacist hesitancy. Of course, this conversation must be private, in a designated counseling area that is physically and psychologically safe for the patient and conducive to an uninterrupted counseling session.

PATIENT MEDICATION COUNSELING QUESTIONS

We suggest that counseling pharmacists engage patients in mutual exchanges of important information about medication needs through the use of several basic questions (see Figure 9.1). These questions are basically the same for any interactive counseling session. The focus of the questioning is *disease specific* with additional emphasis upon the *medication regimen, associative medications effects (e.g., side effects), basic monitoring needs,*

Primary Questions
1. What did your doctor tell you to take the medication for?
2. How did the doctor tell you to take the medication?
3. What did the doctor tell you about side effects, interactions and other warnings about the medication?

Secondary Questions
4. Did the doctor instruct you on how to monitor . . . (describe specific self-monitoring activity)?
5. What do you need to know about refills, missed doses, or proper storage?
6. Miscellaneous questions

FIGURE 9.1. The basic patient medication counseling questions

and refill information. The patient counseling questions are classified as *primary questions* and *secondary questions.* The primary questions should be asked in *all* sessions involving *new* prescription orders. Secondary questions should be asked when the pharmacist, in his or her professional judgment, deems them necessary. Which primary or secondary questions to ask when counseling refill requests can also be determined by the pharmacist.

The first primary question, ''What did your doctor tell you to take the medication for?'' can be elaborated upon, depending on the nature of the therapy, to questions such as, ''What is this medication supposed to do?'' The second question can be expressed in a variety of ways pertaining to the patient or patient's therapy. These ways can include, ''How are you supposed to take this medication?'' or ''How often are you supposed to take this medication?'' or ''How much are you supposed to take?'' or ''How long are you to be on this medication?'' The final primary question can be individualized and expressed as, ''What were some of the bad or good effects of the medication that you were told to expect?'' or ''Were you told by the doctor not to take any other medications at the same time?'' or ''Do you have any specific concerns about taking this medication?''

Secondary questions should be asked to fit the individual nature of the counseling session. Often patients will have the additional responsibility of monitoring some aspect of their therapy. Questions such as, ''Do you know how to take a blood sugar (or blood pressure, pulse, and temperature)?'' or ''Were you told how to use this inhaler (or other machine or apparatus)?'' might be appropriate. Other secondary questions to be asked might be, ''If you were to miss a dose, what were you told to do?'' or ''Do you know how to properly store or put away this medication?'' or ''Do you understand that there are no refills for this prescription medication?''

VERIFICATION OF THE PATIENT COUNSELING SESSION

Verification indicating that the patient understood the questions asked and what had been explained is necessary for successful completion of an interactive patient counseling session. The pharmacist must be convinced that he or she has "gotten the message across" to the patient or caregiver. This adds very little time to the process, and assures that the small amount of time spent during the whole session does not result in ineffectual or less productive patient counseling. The pharmacist may believe that he or she is addressing the problem of verification by simply asking the patient, "Do you understand . . . ?" However, patients often will respond in the affirmative, when that might not be the case, in order to please the pharmacist or to abruptly end the conversation. It is much better to ask the patient to repeat back what has been asked, or to repeat in her or his own words what has been explained. For example, when counseling a diabetic patient on an oral anti-hyperglycemic medication, the pharmacist might ask, "What are you supposed to do if you begin to become sweaty, shaky, or confused because your blood sugar may be too low?" This kind of questioning will provide verification and will also serve to reinforce better medication compliance behavior.

COUNSELING REFILL PRESCRIPTIONS

Counseling refill prescriptions is just as important. The counseling session for refills can reintroduce the primary and secondary questions previously asked. However, this session should also address any changes or alterations of medication therapy that may have occurred since the original prescription was filled or the last refill dispensed. These changes will have to be noted and documented. Perhaps the dose of an anti-hypertensive medication has to be changed because the doctor was not getting the expected patient response. A refill counseling session may determine that the patient was not taking the medication correctly. The reuse of the primary and secondary questions for refill counseling will also reaffirm that the patient continues to take the medication correctly for the proper reasons. In addition, any new concerns about undesirable medication effects can be resolved.

SCENARIO DEVELOPMENT

The application of patient medication counseling skills to any community-based pharmacy practice setting still must be designed to fulfill

TABLE 9.1. Twelve Steps to Successful Patient Counseling.

1. Provide an area for maintaining privacy during counseling.
2. Express concern for and interest in the patient or caregiver.
3. Assess patient's prior knowledge of the disease/treatment.
4. Display appropriate non-verbal behaviors.
5. Use language the patient can understand.
6. Maintain control and direction of the counseling session.
7. Make use of appropriate patient medication profile information.
8. Ask the primary questions and appropriate secondary questions and elicit the patient's response.
9. Utilize the prescription label's directions for use to assist in presenting the facts and concepts in a logical, sequential order.
10. Summarize the information presented.
11. Determine if the patient understood what has been presented.
12. Keep all information and discussion confidential.

individual practitioner needs. Thus, what follows is a set of realistic patient medication counseling scenarios to reflect actual counseling situations in the pharmacy. They are intended to allow the pharmacist to take part in patient medication counseling activities almost immediately. These scenarios are basic examples of counseling opportunities using routine prescription-filling requests for common disease or symptomatic conditions. They are designed to be easily adaptable to any situation described in each scenario and to be of most use when the scenario format is followed as closely as possible. The format reflects what is suggested for successful patient counseling by the twelve steps to successful counseling (see Table 9.1) and utilizes the basic patient medication counseling questions (Figure 9.1).

CHAPTER 10

Applying Patient Counseling to the Practice Setting (Scenarios)

SCENARIO FORMAT (HOW TO USE A SCENARIO)

Each scenario describes a situation in which a patient brings a prescription(s) into the pharmacy for the treatment of a common disease or symptomatic condition. These scenarios are designed to be easily adaptable to any situation similar to the ones described. A major theme emphasized throughout is patient awareness. How the pharmacist counsels the patient will often depend upon what the patient knows about specific aspects of his or her medication therapy. Thus, each scenario allows the pharmacist to counsel correctly, whatever the extent of the patient's awareness. For example, a pharmacist may counsel differently where the patient appears to be unaware of how to take the medication or what are common side effects associated with a medication.

Each scenario has the following format:

a. Patient background
b. Description of the prescription(s) presented
c. Pertinent medication profile information
   1. Past medical history
   2. Allergies
   3. Past and/or current medications
d. The three primary questions
   1. What did your doctor tell you the medication is for?
   2. How did your doctor tell you to take the medication?
   3. What did the doctor tell you about side effects, interactions, and other warnings about this medication?
e. Pertinent secondary questions
   1. Did the doctor tell you how to monitor . . . ?

2. Refill information question(s)
3. Other
4. Suggested prescription label directions for use

A little practice using each scenario is recommended. This format is also adaptable to *other* scenarios, so you can create your own. You *can* be a successful and effective patient medication counselor!

SCENARIO 1: TYPE II (ADULT ONSET) DIABETES

Ms. Smith is a fifty-year-old newly diagnosed diabetic. She occasionally comes to your store for OTC analgesics. She has a prescription for:
Glucotrol® 5 mg. tablets
#120
Take one tablet b.i.d.
No refills

Her pertinent medication profile information reads as follows:
Medical History:
Hypertension
Urinary tract infection
ALLERGIES: None
Past Medications:
Bactrim®, 1 DS tablet b.i.d. (#14)
Hydrochlorothiazide 25 mg. q.d. (#50)
Acetaminophen tablets 500 mg. p.r.n.

1. "WHAT DID YOUR DOCTOR TELL YOU THE MEDICATION IS FOR?"
   (a) **Patient is aware of indication:** Ms. Smith informs the pharmacist that she is taking Glucotrol® to control her blood sugar.
   (b) **Patient is unaware of indication:** Ms. Smith replies that "the doctor told me to take this tablet twice a day and come back and see him in two months." The pharmacist suggests, "Ms. Smith, this prescription is for Glucotrol®, a tablet you can take by mouth in order to control your blood sugar."
2. "HOW DID YOUR DOCTOR TELL YOU TO TAKE THE MEDICA-TION?"
   (a) **Patient is aware of medication regimen:** Ms. Smith replies, "I am to take one tablet twice a day," and the pharmacist verifies this by

reviewing the prescription label directions[1] with the patient and adds, "It's important to take these at evenly spaced intervals like 8 a.m. and 8 p.m. and 1/2 hour before eating to get the maximum benefits of the drug. Remember, follow the directions on the label."

(b) **Patient is unaware of drug regimen:** Ms. Smith replies, "I'm not sure; I think I take one twice a day, but I'm not sure how long." The pharmacist reviews the prescription label directions[1] with the patient and says, "Yes, you take one of these tablets twice a day at evenly spaced intervals like 8 a.m. and 8 p.m. and 1/2 hour before eating. This will give you the maximum benefit of the medication."

3. "WHAT DID THE DOCTOR TELL YOU ABOUT SIDE EFFECTS, INTERACTIONS, AND OTHER WARNINGS ABOUT THIS MEDICATION?"

(a) **Patient is aware of side effects, etc.:** Ms. Smith responds, "The doctor told me about the possibility of having abnormally low blood sugars and that I could counteract it with some hard candy or fruit juice. He also told me this medicine may be affected by sulfa drugs or alcohol. He also suggested that my blood pressure pill may interfere with blood sugar control, but this will show in my blood sugars I check." The pharmacist replies, "OK, and one of the medications that you took recently for a urinary tract infection, Bactrim®, is a sulfa drug. It is important that you relay this information to any other doctors you may have. Also, if you take your Glucotrol® with alcohol, it may cause an uncomfortable flushing sensation, associated with headache, nausea, and stomach upset."

(b) **Patient is unaware of side effects, etc.:** "No, he just told me to call if I had problems and see him again in two months." The pharmacist tells Ms. Smith that Glucotrol® has few side effects but here are some things you should know about them:

1. "It's important that you do not skip a meal and do eat at regular intervals. If you begin to become sweaty, shaky, confused, or anxious due to low blood sugar, and an overall feeling of 'impending doom,' you should take 1/2 cup of fruit juice or a couple of pieces of hard candy (keep them handy) to raise your blood sugar. Also, that would be a good time to check your blood sugar to see if it is low. If this happens often, you should notify the doctor."

2. "There is a potential for medication interactions with the Bactrim® you took in the past and your Glucotrol® pill, so you

[1]Take one tablet by mouth twice a day 1/2 hour before breakfast and 1/2 hour before dinner until next doctor's visit for blood sugar.

should check your blood sugar level as needed to control it. Check with your doctor if you have trouble with these medications or any others. Also, don't drink alcohol with this medicine at any time."

4. "DID THE DOCTOR INSTRUCT YOU HOW TO MONITOR YOUR BLOOD SUGAR?"

   (a) **Patient is aware of self-monitoring techniques:** Ms. Smith replies that she spent several mornings working with a nurse who taught her how to do home blood glucose monitoring and helped her in the selection of an appropriate test kit. "Do you (to the pharmacist) sell supplies for the (name of a particular kit)?"

   (b) **Patient is unaware of self-monitoring techniques:** Ms. Smith replies, "He told me just to ask at the pharmacy." The pharmacist offers, "I have a wide variety of kits available, depending on how much you are willing to spend to make it easier on yourself to improve the accuracy of your blood sugar measurements. You will need to prick your finger to get a drop of blood and place it on a special strip like this (pharmacist reviews instructions on how to monitor blood sugar levels with the patient using the materials from the appropriate kit). You will need to do this before each meal and probably at bedtime, and record the times and blood sugar readings in a log book. These numbers will assist your doctor in adjusting the medication if needed."

5. REFILL INFORMATION

   "Ms. Smith, you should see your doctor within two months because there are no refills on the prescription, and he will want to evaluate your response to the medication at that time."

SCENARIO 2: CHRONIC OBSTRUCTIVE PULMONARY DISEASE (COPD)

Mr. Brown is a forty-five-year-old patient who has suffered from COPD for the past year. He has been coming to your pharmacy for most of his medications. He has a new prescription for:

Theodur® 250 mg.
#100
Take one tablet po. b.i.d.
No refills

His pertinent medication profile information includes:
Medical History:
Back Pain

Ulcer
Upper Respiratory Infection
COPD
ALLERGIES: Penicillin
Past Medications:
Motrin® 600 mg. tablets (#20)
Zantac® 150 mg. tablets (#60)
Cipro® 500 mg. tablets (#14)
Current Medications:
Alupent® MDI
Beclovent® MDI

1. "WHAT DID YOUR DOCTOR TELL YOU THE MEDICATION IS FOR?"
   (a) **Patient is aware of indication:** Mr. Brown informs the pharmacist that he will be taking theophylline to assist him with breathing.
   (b) **Patient is unaware of indication:** Mr. Brown states, "The doctor told me to take these tablets; I think he said it was for breathing." The pharmacist replies, "Mr. Brown, this prescription is for Theodur®, a theophylline preparation that you can take by mouth to help you breath easier."
2. "HOW DID YOUR DOCTOR TELL YOU TO TAKE THE MEDICATION?"
   (a) **Patient is aware of medication regimen:** Mr. Brown replies, "I am to take one tablet twice a day, but I need to come back and see him in a week." The pharmacist reviews the prescription label directions[2] with the patient and suggests, "It's important to take these tablets at evenly spaced intervals like 8 a.m. and 8 p.m. to receive the maximum benefits from the medication and help minimize any side effects. Keep taking them this way until the doctor tells you to stop. Remember to follow the directions on the label."
   (b) **Patient is unaware of drug regimen:** Mr. Brown replies, "I'm not sure. I understand that I should take one twice a day, but I don't know when I can stop taking this medication." The pharmacist reviews the prescription label directions[2] with the patient and says, "Yes, you take one of these tablets at evenly spaced intervals like 8 a.m. and 8 p.m. Keep taking the medication until you see the doctor and he tells you to stop. This will give you the maximum benefit of the medication, and help minimize any side effects."

---

[2]Take one tablet by mouth twice a day at 8 a.m. and 8 p.m. until told to stop for easier breathing.

3. ``WHAT DID THE DOCTOR TELL YOU ABOUT SIDE EFFECTS, INTERACTIONS, AND OTHER WARNINGS ABOUT THIS MEDICATION?``

    (a) **Patient is aware of side effects, etc.:** Mr. Brown responds, ``The doctor told me about the possibility of nervousness, irritability and frequent urination. If I have an increase in my heart rate, breathing rate or frequent vomiting, I am to contact him immediately. The pharmacist responds, ``Good, now I see that you had a previous prescription for an antibiotic known as Cipro® which should not always be taken with theophylline. You should advise all doctors you may see that you are on Theodur®, because of the potential of it interacting with Cipro® or other medications. Many over-the-counter medications may interact with theophylline. Also, drinking coffee, tea and colas, and smoking cigarettes can affect the action of theophylline. You should tell your doctor if you change your use of these substances.``

    (b) **Patient is unaware of side effects, etc.:** ``No, he just told me to call if I had any problems and see him in a week.`` The pharmacist informs Mr. Brown that Theodur® has some side effects that he should be aware of:

    1. Nausea, vomiting, stomach pain, abdominal cramps or lack of appetite. Take this medication with meals or with an antacid or with a full glass of liquid.

    2. It is possible that the medication may cause nervousness, irritability and frequent urination. If these effects persist, contact your doctor.

    3. If you have any increase in your heart rate, breathing rate or frequent vomiting, or seizures contact your doctor immediately.

    ``I see that you had a previous prescription for an antibiotic known as Cipro® which should not always be taken with theophylline. You should advise all doctors that you may see you are on Theodur®, because of the potential of it interacting with Cipro® and with other medications. Many over-the-counter medications may interact with theophylline. Also, drinking coffee, tea and colas, and smoking cigarettes can affect the action of theophylline. You should tell your doctor if you change your use of these substances.``

4. REFILL INFORMATION

    (a) ``Mr. Brown, remember to see your doctor in a week. If he wants you to continue taking this medication, you will have enough for six more weeks because there are no refills on this prescription. He may want to evaluate you at that time.``

    (b) (If Mr. Brown had not been asked to see the doctor in a week, the pharmacist might respond as follows): ''Mr. Brown, you should see your doctor in six weeks, if not before then, because there are no refills on this prescription. He may want to evaluate your response at that time.''

SCENARIO 3: HYPERTENSION

Mr. Smith is a forty-three-year-old patient who has just been diagnosed with hypertension. His family has been coming to your pharmacy for the past five years. He has a new prescription for:
Tenormin® 50 mg.
#60
Take one tablet every day
No refills

His pertinent medication profile information shows:
Medical History:
Pharyngitis
Ulcer
Sleeplessness
ALLERGIES: None
Past Medications:
Polymox® 250 mg. capsules (#21) (for sinus infection)
Zantac® 150 mg. tablets (#60) (for ulcer)
Diazepam® 2 mg. tablets (#15) (for agitation)

1. ''WHAT DID YOUR DOCTOR TELL YOU THE MEDICATION IS FOR?''
   (a) **Patient is aware of indication:** Mr. Smith informs the pharmacist that he will be taking Tenormin® to control his blood pressure.
   (b) **Patient is unaware of indication:** Mr. Smith states, ''The doctor told me to take one of these tablets a day and to come back and see him in two months.'' The pharmacist responds, ''Mr. Smith, these Tenormin® tablets will help control your blood pressure.''
2. ''HOW DID YOUR DOCTOR TELL YOU TO TAKE THE MEDICA-TION?''
   (a) **Patient is aware of medication regimen:** Mr. Smith replies, ''I am to take one of these tablets a day, and come back and see him in two months.'' The pharmacist reviews the prescription label directions[3]

---

[3]Take one tablet by mouth every day at 10 a.m. until told to stop for high blood pressure.

with the patient and tells Mr. Smith, "You have just enough tablets for two months until your appointment. It's important that you continue to keep taking these tablets unless the physician advises you otherwise."

(b) **Patient is unaware of drug regimen:** Mr. Smith replies, "I'm not sure; I know I am to take one tablet a day, but I don't know when I can stop taking the medication." The pharmacist reviews the prescription label directions[3] with the patient and tells Mr. Smith, "You have just enough tablets for two months until you have your next appointment. It's important that you continue to keep taking these tablets unless the physician advises you otherwise."

3. "WHAT DID THE DOCTOR TELL YOU ABOUT SIDE EFFECTS, INTERACTIONS, AND OTHER WARNINGS ABOUT THIS MEDICATION?"

(a) **Patient is aware of side effects, etc.:** "The doctor told me not to get up too quickly so as to avoid becoming dizzy or lightheaded. He also told me that this medication will decrease the rate of my heartbeat." The pharmacist agrees and responds, "In addition, it is important not to abruptly stop taking the medication because of the potential for initiating 'rebound hypertension.' "

(b) **Patient is unaware of side effects:** "No, he just told me to call if I had any problems and to see him in two months." The pharmacist informs Mr. Smith that Tenormin® has some common side effects he should be aware of:

1. A decrease in heart rate; check pulse daily before taking the tablet. If your pulse rate is less than sixty beats per minute, then you should contact the doctor before taking the next tablet.

2. A feeling of dizziness or lightheadedness may occur if you get up too quickly from sitting or lying down. If this occurs, you should take your time before standing.

3. Do not stop taking the medication without consulting your physician. It is important that you keep your appointment in two months.

4. "DID THE DOCTOR INSTRUCT YOU HOW TO MONITOR YOUR BLOOD PRESSURE AND PULSE?"

(a) **Patient is aware of self-monitoring techniques:** Mr. Smith replies, "The doctor told me the medication could decrease my heart rate, and I should check my pulse daily before taking the tablet. If my pulse rate is less than sixty beats per minute, then I will contact him (the doctor) before taking my next dose. My doctor suggested that I should investigate purchasing a blood pressure cuff. Do you sell these?" "Why, yes," the pharmacist responds. "We have several different types according to how much money you wish to spend. I can show you how to work them. I also suggest that you check your blood pressure daily."

(b) **Patient is unaware of self-monitoring techniques:** Mr. Smith replies, "He told me just to ask at the pharmacy." The pharmacist responds, "There are two things you should monitor while taking this medication. The first is your pulse because the medication can decrease your heart rate. You should check your pulse daily before taking your next dose. If your pulse is less than sixty beats per minute, then you should contact your doctor before taking your next dose. Secondly, it would be helpful to monitor your blood pressure to evaluate your response to your medication. I suggest two options. We have an automated device over there in the corner of the store that you can use free of charge during any visit to our store. Or you may purchase a blood pressure cuff of your own. We have several models available depending on how much you may wish to spend. You should monitor your blood pressure daily or three times a week during a peaceful time in your day. It would be helpful if you kept a record of these pressures to assist your physician in adjusting your dose."

5. REFILL INFORMATION
"Mr. Smith, you should be sure to see your doctor within two months because there are no refills on the prescription. It is very important that you do not run out of tablets."

SCENARIO 4: URINARY TRACT INFECTION

Jane Doe is a twenty-eight-year-old female who has been coming to your pharmacy for the past five years. She has a long history of asthma. She recently has experienced burning and frequent urination. She visited her gynecologist and brings the following prescription to you:

Cipro® 250 mg. tablets
#14
Take one tablet twice daily
No refills

Her pertinent medication profile information is as follows:
Medical History:
Asthma
ALLERGIES: PCN, Codeine, Sulfa
Past Medications:
Ortho Novum®, take as directed (last refill three months ago)

Proventil® MDI (last refill six months ago)

Theodur® 200 mg. t.i.d. (last refill one year ago)

1. "WHAT DID YOUR DOCTOR TELL YOU THE MEDICATION IS FOR?"
   (a) **Patient is aware of indication:** Ms. Doe informs the pharmacist that she knows this is an antibiotic for her urinary tract infection.
   (b) **Patient is unaware of indication:** Ms. Doe states, "The doctor told me to take a tablet twice a day and to call him at the end of the week." The pharmacist responds, "This is an antibiotic to treat your urinary tract infection."

2. "HOW DID YOUR DOCTOR TELL YOU TO TAKE THE MEDICATION?"
   (a) **Patient is aware of medication regimen:** Ms. Doe replies, "I am to take a tablet twice a day until they are all gone." The pharmacist reviews the prescription label directions[4] with her and tells Ms. Doe, "That is correct; even though your symptoms may disappear, it is important to complete all the medication."
   (b) **Patient is unaware of medication regimen:** Ms. Doe replies, "I'm supposed to take one tablet twice a day, but I don't know for how long." The pharmacist reviews the prescription label directions[4] with her and tells Ms. Doe, "Yes, you should take these twice a day, and it is important that you finish them, even though your symptoms may disappear within a day or two."

3. "WHAT DID THE DOCTOR TELL YOU ABOUT SIDE EFFECTS, INTERACTIONS, AND OTHER WARNINGS ABOUT THIS MEDICATION?"
   (a) **Patient is aware of side effects, etc.:** "The doctor told me the medication may upset my stomach and he encouraged me to take it with meals. He (the doctor) also suggests the possibility of headaches, restlessness or a skin rash." The pharmacist agrees and responds, "In addition it is very important not to take this medicine while you are pregnant. I see from your history that you have taken Theodur® in the past. Are you still taking this medication?" Ms. Doe replies, "No, I haven't had problems with my asthma lately. If I do I've been advised to use my Proventil® Inhaler." The pharmacist responds, "That's good because there is a drug interaction between this antibiotic and the Theodur®. If you begin taking the Theodur® again within the next week, you should consult with your physician to recommend an alternative antibiotic to avoid the interaction."

[4]Take one tablet by mouth twice a day at 8 a.m. and 6 p.m. with meals until gone for urinary tract infection.

(b) **Patient is unaware of side effects, etc.:** "No, he just told me to call if I had any problems." The pharmacist informs Ms. Doe that Cipro® has a number of side effects she should be aware of:

1. To avoid stomach upset, you should take it with meals.
2. Headaches
3. Restlessness
4. Skin rash
5. In addition it is very important not to take this medicine while you are pregnant.

I see by your medication history that you have taken Theodur® in the past. Are you still taking this medication?" Ms. Doe replies, "No, I haven't had problems with my asthma lately. If I do I've been advised to use my Proventil® Inhaler." The pharmacist responds, "That's good because there is a drug interaction between this antibiotic and the Theodur®. If you begin taking the Theodur® again within the next week, you should consult the doctor to recommend an alternative antibiotic to avoid the interaction."

4. "DID THE DOCTOR INSTRUCT YOU HOW TO MONITOR YOUR INFECTION?"

   (a) **Patient is aware of self-monitoring techniques:** "The doctor told me my symptoms should go away in a few days, but to continue taking the medication. If I was not any better, I was to contact him."

   (b) **Patient is unaware of self-monitoring techniques:** "The doctor told me to call if I didn't feel better after I had finished the medicine." The pharmacist responds, "It should only take a short time for your symptoms to go away. However it is important that you finish all the tablets."

5. REFILL INFORMATION
   Ms. Doe, there are no refills on this prescription.

SCENARIO 5: CHEMOPROPHYLAXIS FOR INFECTIVE ENDOCARDITIS

Mr. Bob Anderson is a thirty-two-year-old patient. He sporadically comes to your pharmacy for refill medications. He has told you that he was diagnosed years ago with mitral valve prolapse. He has a new prescription for:

Polymox® 500 mg. tablets
#18
Take six capsules before and three capsules after teeth cleaning.
Refill X 4

His pertinent medication profile information reads as follows:

Medical History:

Tooth removal

Anxiety

ALLERGIES: None

Past Medications:

Motrin® 600 mg. (#15) (for joint pain)

Ativan® 1 mg. tablets (#20) (for restlessness)

1. "WHAT DID YOUR DOCTOR TELL YOU THE MEDICATION IS FOR?"

   (a) **Patient is aware of medication indication:** Mr. Anderson informs the pharmacist that he will be taking the antibiotic, prior to having his teeth cleaned, to prevent any bacteria from infecting his bloodstream since he was recently diagnosed with mitral valve prolapse.

   (b) **Patient is unaware of medication indication:** Mr. Anderson states, "The doctor told me to take these before I go to the dentist to have my teeth cleaned." The pharmacist adds, "This antibiotic will prevent any bacteria from infecting your bloodstream. Since you have mitral valve prolapse, you have an increased risk for an infection in your heart."

2. "HOW DID YOUR DOCTOR TELL YOU TO TAKE THE MEDICA-TION?"

   (a) **Patient is aware of medication regimen:** Mr. Anderson replies, "I am to take six capsules before I go to have my teeth cleaned, and then three capsules afterwards." The pharmacist reviews the prescription label directions[5] with the patient and tells Mr. Anderson, "You should have enough of these capsules for two visits."

   (b) **Patient is unaware of medication regimen:** Mr. Anderson replies, "I'm not sure; he just told me to follow the directions of the label." The pharmacist reviews the prescription label directions[5] with the patient and tells Mr. Anderson, "You should take six capsules one hour before having your teeth cleaned, and then take three capsules six hours after the first dose. There's enough in the bottle for two dentist visits."

3. "WHAT DID THE DOCTOR TELL YOU ABOUT SIDE EFFECTS, INTERACTIONS, AND OTHER WARNINGS ABOUT THIS MEDICATION?"

   (a) **Patient is aware of side effects:** "The doctor told me that this could

---

[5]Take six (6) capsules by mouth one hour before teeth cleaning and three (3) capsules 6 hours after the first dose with a big glass of water to prevent heart infection.

make me queasy. If so, I should eat a snack like crackers or toast before I take the medication." The pharmacist agrees and responds, "In addition, it would be helpful to take these capsules with a big glass of water."

(b) **Patient is unaware of side effects:** "No, he did not." The pharmacist responds, "These capsules may make you a little queasy. If so, you may eat some crackers or drink some milk before taking the medication. It would be helpful if you took these capsules with a big glass of water."

4. REFILL INFORMATION

Mr. Anderson, you have enough capsules in the vial for two dentist visits. In other words, if you see the dentist twice a year this should last for a year. However, if you need additional medication you have four refills on this prescription.

SCENARIO 6: MENOPAUSE

Mrs. Smith is a forty-seven-year-old woman who has been having sudden feelings of warmth and skin flushing for the past month. She recently has complaints of waking at night drenched with perspiration. She has not had a menstrual period for the past seven months. Following her visit to her gynecologist, she comes to your pharmacy with the following prescriptions:

Premarin® 0.3 mg. tablets
#75
Take one tablet daily.
Provera® 5 mg. tablets
#30
Take one tablet daily, day 1 to day 10 of every month only.

Her pertinent medication profile information is as follows:
Medical History:
Duodenal ulcer (six years ago)
ALLERGIES: None
Past Medications:
Zantac® 150 mg. tablets (#60) (for ulcer)
Diazepam 2 mg. tablets (#15) (for anxiety)

1. "WHAT DID YOUR DOCTOR TELL YOU THE MEDICATION IS FOR?"
   a. **Patient is aware of indication:** Mrs. Smith informs the pharmacist that she will be taking this combination to help with the hot flashes

she has been experiencing the past seven months. The pharmacist agrees and adds that the medication should help prevent osteoporosis (bone weakening) and atherosclerosis (hardening of the arteries).

b. **Patient is unaware of indication:** Mrs. Smith states, "The doctor told me to take each one of these tablets as described on the pill bottle and to come back and see him in two months." The pharmacist responds, "Mrs. Smith, these tablets are used to help reduce the occurrence of hot flashes, bone weakening and hardening of the arteries that occurs in women who are going through the change of life."

2. "HOW DID YOUR DOCTOR TELL YOU TO TAKE THE MEDICATION?"

a. **Patient is aware of medication regimen:** Mrs. Smith replies, "I am to take one Premarin® tablet every day and the Provera® only for the first ten days of each month." The pharmacist reviews the prescription label directions[6] with the patient and tells Mrs. Smith, "Try to take the tablets at the same time every day so that you don't forget to take a dose. You have just enough tablets for three months."

b. **Patient is unaware of drug regimen:** Mrs. Smith replies, "I'm not sure. I know I am to take one tablet a day of each prescription but I don't know for how long." The pharmacist reviews the prescription label directions[6] with the patient and tells Mrs. Smith, "You should take the one Premarin® (the green tablet) every day and the Provera® (the white tablet) every day only for the first ten days of each month. Try to take the tablets at the same time every day so that you don't forget to take a dose. You have just enough tablets for three months."

3. "WHAT DID THE DOCTOR TELL YOU ABOUT THE SIDE EFFECTS, INTERACTIONS AND OTHER WARNINGS ABOUT THIS MEDICATION?"

a. **Patient is aware of side effects, etc.:** "The doctor explained to me the Premarin® may cause some nausea, cramps, bloating, diarrhea or weight and appetite changes. I may retain water or have black or brown skin patches appear on my skin. I should contact him immediately if I suffer from a severe headache, alteration in vision, numbness, or sharp chest pain." The pharmacist responds, "You may take these with food to help minimize any nausea." The pharmacist continues by inquiring, "What effects did your doctor tell you regarding the Provera®?" Mrs. Smith responds, "They have similar side effects, but the Provera® may also cause depression."

---

[6](Premarin®) Take one tablet by mouth daily at 10 a.m. until next doctor visit for hot flashes. (Provera®) Take one tablet by mouth daily at 10 a.m. first ten days of the month until next doctor visit for hot flashes.

The pharmacist agrees and adds, ''Both medications may increase the risk of strokes, high blood pressure, blood clots, or heart attacks. You should not smoke cigarettes because this will add to the risk of causing these serious conditions. Here's some written product information to explain more about the risks associated with Premarin® and Provera®.''

b. **Patient is unaware of side effects:** The pharmacist asks, ''Did the doctor tell you to look for any unwanted side effects associated with these medications?'' Mrs. Smith replies, ''No, he just told me to call if I had any problems and to see him in three months.'' The pharmacist informs Mrs. Smith that Premarin® has some commonly occurring side effects she should be aware of:

   1. Nausea, cramps, bloating, diarrhea or some weight and appetite changes. Taking these with food will help to minimize any nausea.
   2. Fluid retention
   3. Black or brown skin patches
   4. Contact the doctor immediately if you suffer from a severe headache, alteration in vision, numbness or sharp chest pain.

   ''The Provera® may cause similar side effects, but in addition may cause depression. Both medications may increase the risk of strokes, blood clots, high blood pressure, blood clots, or heart attacks. You should not smoke cigarettes because this will add to the risk of causing these serious conditions. Here's some written product information to explain more about the risks associated with Premarin® and Provera®.''

4. ''DID THE DOCTOR INSTRUCT YOU ON OTHER WAYS TO MINIMIZE THE OCCURRENCE OF OSTEOPOROSIS (BONE WEAKENING)?''

   a. **Patient is aware of prevention:** The pharmacist asks, ''Did the doctor tell you to take any calcium supplements?'' Mrs. Smith responds, ''Yes, we discussed that I should be getting one gram of calcium daily, either through diet or supplements. Could you recommend a calcium supplement?'' The pharmacist agrees, and assists in the selection of an over-the-counter calcium supplement.

   b. **Patient is unaware of prevention:** The pharmacist asks, ''Did the doctor tell you to take any calcium supplements?'' Mrs. Smith responds, ''No, he told me these pills would help with my problems.'' The pharmacist replies, ''Be sure to check with the doctor, but you should be taking one gram of calcium daily, either through diet or supplements. The average daily intake is about 500 mg. of calcium. I recommend that you choose from any of several calcium supplements that could provide the additional amount you may need."

5. REFILL INFORMATION

"Mrs. Smith, there are no refills on these prescriptions. But there is enough medication to last for three months. Be sure to see your doctor before you run out. Until then it is important that you continue to take the medications as directed on the prescription label."

SCENARIO 7: PAIN MANAGEMENT

Susan Spicer is a fifty-five-year-old female who occasionally visits your pharmacy. She comes to your pharmacy with her husband after being discharged from the hospital. During her hospital stay she was found to have bone cancer. She has the following prescription to be filled:

MS Contin® 60 mg. tablets.
#60
Take one tablet twice a day.
No refills

Her pertinent medication profile information reads as follows:

Medical History:
Lumbar Laminectomy (two years ago)
Hysterectomy (ten years ago)
Hypertension
ALLERGIES: Sulfa

Current Medications:
Atenolol® 50 mg. q.d.
Premarin® 0.3 mg. tabs UTD

Past Medications:
Amoxicillin® 250 mg. t.i.d.
Tagamet® 300 mg. q. h.s.
Diazepam 2 mg. tablets. p.r.n.

1. "WHAT DID YOUR DOCTOR TELL YOU THE MEDICATION IS FOR?"

   a. **Patient is aware of indication:** Mrs. Spicer tells the pharmacist, "This is to relieve my bone pain and keep me comfortable. I think these are the same pills the doctor started me on in the hospital to take the place of morphine injections." The pharmacist agrees and adds, "These tablets are long acting and should help control your pain over a long period of time."

   b. **Patient is unaware of indication:** Mrs. Spicer tells the pharmacist,

"I think these pills are supposed to relieve my bone pain and keep me comfortable. But are they strong enough?" "Don't worry," replies the pharmacist. "These tablets are strong enough for the severest pain. They are probably the same tablets that the doctor started giving to you in the hospital to take the place of the pain-relieving injections. These are long-acting and should help to control your pain over an extended period of time."

2. "HOW DID YOUR DOCTOR TELL YOU TO TAKE THE MEDICA-TION?"

   a. **Patient is aware of medication regimen:** Mrs. Spicer replies, "I am to take one tablet every twelve hours." The pharmacist reviews the prescription label directions[7] with the patient and offers, "That's correct. It is important that you take these tablets on regularly scheduled hours, like at 8 a.m. and 8 p.m., rather than after the pain starts. If you do so, you will keep a constant blood level of pain medication and prevent the pain from coming back. You can also supplement these with some over-the-counter Tylenol® (acet-aminophen) or Nuprin® (ibuprofen), if necessary."

   b. **Patient is unaware of medication regimen:** Mrs. Spicer replies, "The doctor told me I could take these twice a day as needed for pain, but I don't want to become addicted to this medicine." The pharmacist reviews the prescription label directions[7] with the patient and offers, "If your physician prescribed this medication for you, it is because you need a strong analgesic for your pain, and she is not concerned with addiction, and neither should you be. The purpose of this medication is to keep you from having any severe pain; therefore, it is important that you take these tablets regularly rather than wait for the pain to start. If you take these tablets on a timely basis, like at 8 a.m. and 8 p.m., you will keep a constant blood level of pain medication. You may also supplement these with some over-the-counter pain-reliever like Tylenol® (acetaminophen) or Advil® (ibuprofen), if necessary."

3. "WHAT DID THE DOCTOR TELL YOU ABOUT SIDE EFFECTS, INTERACTIONS AND OTHER WARNINGS ABOUT THIS MEDICATION?"

   a. **Patient is aware of side effects, etc.:** "The doctor told me the medication may make me drowsy or sleepy and I should not drive nor drink while I am taking it. She said I may get an upset stomach or constipation." The pharmacist responds, "To help minimize any

---

[7]Take one tablet by mouth twice a day (at 8 a.m. and 8 p.m. to start) for thirty days to prevent severe pain.

queasiness you should lie down or sit quietly for a while after taking the tablet. I suggest taking a stool softener daily to help prevent constipation. If you have any difficulty breathing, you should notify a family member to contact your doctor immediately. Also, I see from your medication profile you had a prescription filled for Valium® some time ago. It's important that you do not use it with the MS Contin because it may increase the side effects."

b. **Patient is unaware of side effects, etc.:** Mrs. Spicer responds, "The doctor told me not to drive or drink while on this medication." The pharmacist agrees and offers, "It may make you nauseous or constipated. To help minimize any queasiness you should lie down or sit quietly for a while after taking the tablet. I suggest taking a stool softener daily to help prevent constipation. If you have any difficulty breathing, you should notify a family member to contact your doctor immediately. Also, I see from your medication profile you had a prescription filled for Valium® some time ago. It's important that you do not use it with the MS Contin because it may increase the side effects."

4. "DID THE DOCTOR TELL YOU HOW TO MONITOR THE PAIN-RELIEVING EFFECTS OF THE MEDICATION?"

a. **Patient is aware of monitoring the effects:** Mrs. Spicer responds, "She (the doctor) told me that I will continue to have adequate relief with this dose of Morphine for awhile, but that I might become tolerant to its pain-relieving effects. If this occurs she wants me to contact her and we can discuss altering the dose." The pharmacist responds, "These type of tablets can be easily changed to be given on different timing schedules in order to maintain pain control. But your physician will help you with these adjustments, so do not adjust them on your own."

b. **Patient is unaware of monitoring the effects:** Mrs. Spicer responds, "She simply told me this medication should continue to relieve my pain, and to contact her otherwise." The pharmacist responds, "You should have adequate pain relief; however, you can become tolerant to its pain-relieving effects after a while. If this occurs, you should contact your physician to make the appropriate adjustments. These type of tablets are easily adjustable to different dosage schedules, but do not adjust them on your own."

5. REFILL INFORMATION

"Mrs. Spicer, there are no refills on this prescription. If the doctor wants you to have more of this medication, someone will have to get a new prescription. I can't just get a refill for you over the telephone, so don't wait until you run out. When your doctor does write a new prescription for you, I will be glad to assist you with it as quickly as possible."

SCENARIO 8: ARTHRITIS

Mary Brown is a sixty-eight-year-old female who has been coming to your pharmacy for years. For the past few weeks she has been complaining of fatigue, pain and stiffness when she wakes up. Her hands and wrists appear swollen and she is not able to move them as freely as before. She comes to your pharmacy with the following prescription:

Anaprox® 275 mg. tablets
#90
Take one tablet p.o. t.i.d.
Refill X 2

Her pertinent medication profile information reads as follows:

Medical History:
Diabetes
Hypercholesterolemia
ALLERGIES: Penicillin
Current Medications:
Orinase® 250 mg. p.o. b.i.d. (Diabetes, Type II)
Lopid® 600 mg. tablets p.o. b.i.d. (Hypercholesterolemia)
Past Medications:
Cipro® 500 mg. tablets (for upper respiratory tract infection)
Tylenol #3® tablets (as needed for pain)
Xanax® 0.25 mg. (for sleep)

1. "WHAT DID YOUR DOCTOR TELL YOU THE MEDICATION IS FOR?"
   a. **Patient is aware of indication:** Mrs. Brown tells the pharmacist, "The doctor told me this will help me with my arthritis." The pharmacist agrees and adds, "This medication will help with your pain, swelling and stiffness."
   b. **Patient is unaware of indication:** Mrs. Brown responds, "I think it's for my arthritis." The pharmacist adds, "Yes, this medication will help with the pain, swelling and stiffness associated with your arthritis."
2. "HOW DID YOUR DOCTOR TELL YOU TO TAKE THE MEDICATION?"
   a. **Patient is aware of medication regimen:** Mrs. Brown replies, "I am to take these tablets three times a day." The pharmacist reviews the prescription label directions[8] with the patient and suggests, "The

---

[8]Take one tablet by mouth three times a day at 7 a.m., 2 p.m. and 10 p.m. with food or milk for one full month for arthritis.

Anaprox® should be taken at mealtime or with milk to minimize any stomach irritation. You may also take these with an antacid like Maalox® to prevent any additional irritation to your stomach. Also try to remember to take these tablets at about eight-hour intervals, like 7 a.m., 2 p.m., and 10 p.m., to get the most relief."

    b. **Patient is unaware of medication regimen:** Mrs. Brown replies, "The doctor told me to take these three times a day, but I'm not sure for how long." The pharmacist reviews the prescription label directions[8] with the patient and responds, "It is important that you take the Anaprox® tablets at a time when you can have food, milk or an antacid like Maalox® to prevent any stomach upset. You should continue to take these tablets on a regular basis every day at about eight-hour intervals such as 7 a.m. (with breakfast), 2 p.m., and 10 p.m. (with a snack)."

3. "WHAT DID THE DOCTOR TELL YOU ABOUT SIDE EFFECTS, INTERACTIONS, AND OTHER WARNINGS ABOUT THIS MEDICATION?"

    a. **Patient is aware of side effects, etc.:** Mrs. Brown responds, "The doctor told me I may experience some constipation, nausea or heartburn." The pharmacist replies, "Of course, taking the medicine with food, milk, or antacid will help minimize some of those effects. Also, if you become persistently drowsy, dizzy or have a severe headache you should contact your doctor. Also, this medication has the potential to promote bleeding, therefore it is important that you tell any doctor that you are on this medication. So don't ever take this medication with aspirin. If you need any additional pain relief, you can take Tylenol® (acetaminophen)."

    b. **Patient is unaware of side effects, etc.:** Mrs. Brown responds, "No, he did not offer any other suggestions." The pharmacist responds, "Remember, the Anaprox® won't cause stomach upset or constipation if you take it with food, milk or antacids. Also, if you become persistently drowsy, dizzy or have a severe headache you should contact your doctor. In addition, these drugs have the potential to promote bleeding, so it is important that you tell any doctor that you are on this medication. Remember never to take this medication with aspirin. If you need any additional pain relief you can take Tylenol® (acetaminophen)."

4. "DID YOUR DOCTOR TELL YOU HOW TO MONITOR THE DESIRED EFFECTS OF THE MEDICATION?"

    a. **Patient is aware of monitoring the desired effects:** Mrs. Brown replies, "He (the doctor) told me these tablets should help with my pain, swelling and stiffness. He also told me it may take a couple of weeks before I may begin to feel the effects. He wants me to contact him in a month if I'm not getting enough relief from these tablets." The pharmacist offers, "You should have enough tablets for a full month's trial."

b. **Patient is unaware of monitoring the effects:** Mrs. Brown replies, "He (the doctor) told me to contact him if I did not feel better in three to four weeks." The pharmacist suggests, "You should get relief from the pain, swelling and stiffness in a couple of weeks. However you should continue to take these tablets for a full month's time and give them a chance to work. If they don't, you should contact your physician and discuss your condition with him. You have enough tablets to last you a month."

5. REFILL INFORMATION

"Mrs. Brown, there are two more refills on this prescription. If you think that your response to this medication is satisfactory by the end of the month, then I will be happy to refill it for you at that time. Would you like us to remind you to refill the Anaprox® when your current supply is about to run out?"

SCENARIO 9: HYPOTHYROIDISM

Ellen Anderson is a twenty-eight-year-old, obese female who has been coming to your store for the past seven years. She has been complaining of fatigue, cold intolerance, and a modest weight gain of twenty pounds. Her physician recently ran "some test," after feeling her neck to be enlarged and suggested that she might be hypothyroid. She comes to your pharmacy with the following prescription:

Synthroid® 0.1 mg.
#30
Take one tablet p.o. q.d.
Refill X 2

Her pertinent medication profile information reads as follows:
Medical History
Appendicitis (five years ago)
Removal of wisdom teeth (six years ago)
ALLERGIES: None
Current Medications: None
Past Medications:
Polymox® 250 mg. capsules (for pharyngitis)
Hycodone® Syrup 100 mL. (for cough)
Percocet® tablets, #20 (for wisdom teeth extraction)

1. "WHAT DID THE DOCTOR TELL YOU THE MEDICATION IS FOR?"

   a. **Patient is aware of indication:** Ms. Anderson responds, "The doctor told me this should help correct my thyroid problem." The pharmacist agrees and adds, "This medication should help reverse your fatigue, cold intolerance and weight gain."

   b. **Patient is unaware of indication:** Ms. Anderson responds, "The doctor told me it should make me feel 'back to normal.' " The pharmacist explains, "This medication is a thyroid replacement used in the treatment of hypothyroidism. Your symptoms are typical of hypothyroidism, and this medication should help to reverse your fatigue, intolerance to cold, and weight gain."

2. "HOW DID YOUR DOCTOR TELL YOU TO TAKE THE MEDICA-TION?"

   a. **Patient is aware of medication regimen:** Ms. Anderson replies, "I am to take one tablet daily until I go back to see her." The pharmacist reviews the prescription label directions[9] with the patient and suggests, "Synthroid® is a medication that you may be taking for the rest of your life, so take it religiously every day unless you are told to change it by the doctor. It's usually a good idea to take it at the same time every day. Your physician should follow your response for many years to come."

   b. **Patient is unaware of medication regimen:** Ms. Anderson replies, "The doctor told me to take one daily, but I'm not sure for how long." The pharmacist reviews the prescription label directions[9] with the patient and suggests, "Synthroid® is a medication that you may be taking for the rest of your life, so take it religiously every day unless you are told to change it by the doctor. It's usually a good idea to take it at the same time every day. Your physician should follow your response for many years to come."

3. "WHAT DID THE DOCTOR TELL YOU ABOUT SIDE EFFECTS, INTERACTIONS, AND OTHER WARNINGS ABOUT THIS MEDICATION?"

   a. **Patient is aware of side effects, etc.:** Ms. Anderson responds, "The doctor told me this medication may cause adverse effects if the dose is too high. Such effects could be a fast heartbeat, nervousness, sweating, shaking, diarrhea, and sensitivity to heat." The pharmacist agrees and suggests, "You should contact your doctor if any of these things happen. Pregnancy or birth control pills can interfere with your laboratory tests, so you should tell your physician if you

[9]Take one tablet by mouth every day at 8 a.m. until told to stop for thyroid problem.

plan on becoming pregnant or take birth control pills. Also because there are several other medicines which may interact with it, you should always tell any physician that you take Synthroid®."

b. **Patient is unaware of side effects, etc.:** Ms. Anderson responds, "The doctor just told me to come back and see him in a month." The pharmacist offers, "The medication can cause several adverse effects if the dose is too high. These effects include increased heart rate, nervousness, sweating, shaking, diarrhea, and sensitivity to heat. You should contact your physician if any of this should happen. Pregnancy or birth control pills can interfere with your laboratory tests, so you should tell your physician if you plan on becoming pregnant or take birth control pills. Also because there are other medicines that may interact with Synthroid®, you should always advise any physician that you are on this medication."

4. " DID YOUR DOCTOR TELL YOU HOW HE PLANS TO MONITOR THE EFFECTS OF THE MEDICATION?"

a. **Patient is aware of monitoring the effects:** Ms. Anderson replies, "The doctor told me to come back in and see him in a month. At that time he plans to draw some blood and evaluate my response to the medication." The pharmacist offers, " It is important that you take these tablets on a regular basis so the test results will be valid. Remember to follow the label directions exactly."

b. **Patient is unaware of monitoring the effects:** Ms. Anderson responds, "No, he (the doctor) just told me to come back and see him in a month." The pharmacist suggests, "The physician will probably draw some blood samples at that time and evaluate your response to the medication. It is important that you take these tablets on a regular basis so that the test results will be valid. Remember to follow the label directions exactly."

5. REFILL INFORMATION

"Ms. Anderson, there are two more refills on this prescription. However, you must still return to the doctor in a month, so I can't refill it unless he instructs you to continue taking this medication. If the doctor does want you to continue, I will be happy to refill it at that time."

SCENARIO 10: HYPERLIPIDEMIA

Mr. Jones is a forty-seven-year-old overweight male who has been monitoring his cholesterol level over the past eight months. His last cholesterol reading was 295 mg./dl. He has been trying a low-cholesterol diet but without any success. Today he comes in with a prescription for:

Mevacor® 20 mg. tablets
#60
Take one tablet p.o. b.i.d.
Refill X 4

His pertinent medication profile information reads as follows:
Medical History:
Hypertension
Diabetes Type II
Ulcer (five years ago)
ALLERGIES: None
Current Medications:
Atenolol® 50 mg. p.o. q.d.
Diabeta® 5 mg. b.i.d.
Past Medications:
Erytabs® 250 mg. p.o. q.i.d.
Zantac® 150 mg. p.o. b.i.d.

1. ``WHAT DID YOUR DOCTOR TELL YOU THE MEDICATION IS FOR?``
   a. **Patient aware of indication:** Mr. Jones informs the pharmacist that he will be taking the Mevacor® to ``lower his cholesterol.``
   b. **Patient is unaware of indication:** Mr. Jones states, ``I think I'm supposed to take these tablets for my cholesterol.`` The pharmacist offers, ``Mevacor® is a medication used to lower serum cholesterol. This medication works with a low-cholesterol, low-fat diet, but it does not replace dietary management of cholesterol.``
2. ``HOW DID YOUR DOCTOR TELL YOU TO TAKE THE MEDICATION?``
   a. **Patient is aware of medication regimen:** Mr. Jones replies, ``I am to take one tablet twice a day.`` The pharmacist reviews the prescription label directions[10] with the patient and suggests, ``Take this medication with your morning and evening meals. It will help to remind you what you're taking them for. Continue to take these tablets unless your physician advises you to stop.``
   b. **Patient is unaware of medication regimen:** Mr. Jones replies, ``I'm not sure. I know I should take one twice a day, but I don't know for how long.`` The pharmacist reviews the prescription label directions[10] with the patient and suggests, ``Take these tablets with your morning and evening meals. It will help to remind you what you are

---

[10]Take one tablet by mouth twice a day with morning and evening meals until told to stop for cholesterol.

taking them for. Continue to take these tablets unless your physician advises you to stop."

3. "WHAT DID THE DOCTOR TELL YOU ABOUT SIDE EFFECTS, INTERACTIONS, AND OTHER WARNINGS ABOUT THIS MEDICATION?"

a. **Patient is aware of side effects, etc.:** Mr. Jones responds, "The doctor told me about possible stomach problems, such as cramps, gas, diarrhea, constipation, or indigestion. If I start having muscle pain or cramps he (the doctor) wants me to contact him immediately." The pharmacist agrees and offers, "Your doctor will want to follow your response to the medication through repeated blood tests. He may also check to see if your liver function is normal. You should also have regular eye examinations. I see that you had a previous prescription for an antibiotic known as erythromycin. You should not mix this antibiotic with Mevacor® because of a drug-drug interaction. Also, I see that you are on Alenolol®, a 'beta-blocker.' You may wish to discuss this medication with your doctor at your next visit. Beta-blockers have been shown to increase triglycerides and lower the HDL, the 'good' cholesterol. In addition, it may interfere with your being aware of having a 'low-blood sugar' reaction from your diabetes pill. The doctor might want to try another medication to treat your hypertension."

b. **Patient is unaware of side effects, etc.:** Mr. Jones responds, "No, he just told me to call him if I had any problems and come back and see him in three months." The pharmacist informs Mr. Jones that Mevacor® has some side effects he should be aware of:

1. Stomach problems, such as cramps, gas, diarrhea, constipation or indigestion

2. Abnormal liver function tests. Your doctor will be monitoring this through periodic blood tests.

3. Eye problems. You should have your eyes examined regularly.

4. Muscle pain or cramps – contact your doctor immediately if you experience any muscle tenderness.

"I see that you had a previous prescrition for an antibiotic known as erythromycin. You should not mix this antibiotic with Mevacor® because of a drug-drug interaction. Also, I see that you are on Atenolol®, a 'beta-blocker.' You may wish to discuss this medication with your doctor at your next visit. Beta-blockers have been shown to increase triglycerides and lower the HDL, the 'good' cholesterol. In addition, beta-blockers may interfere with your being aware of a 'low-blood sugar' reaction from your diabetes pill. The doctor might want to try another medication to treat your hypertension."

4. REFILL INFORMATION

" Mr. Jones, there are four more refills on this prescription, enough for four additional months. After you see your physician in three months, you should inquire about continuing this medication for additional refills. I will be glad to refill your fourth refill or update your present prescription at that time.

SCENARIO 11: PEPTIC ULCER DISEASE

Ms. Sarah Williams is a thirty-three-year-old female who has just started a new career in sales this past year. She cares for two small children as a single parent and has been under additional stress with the recent death of her mother. She recently started complaining of abdominal distress, but found that when she ate the pain dissipated temporarily. She just went to see her physician and comes to your pharmacy with the following prescription:

Zantac® 150 tablets
#60
Take one tablet p.o. twice daily.
Refills X 2

Her pertinent medication profile information reads as follows:

Medical History:
Hysterectomy
Urinary Tract Infection
Current Medications:
Provera® 0.3 mg.
Past Medications:
Macrodantin® 50 mg. p.o. q.i.d.
Tylenol #3®

1. "WHAT DID YOUR DOCTOR TELL YOU THE MEDICATION IS FOR?"
   a. **Patient is aware of indication:** Ms. Williams replies, "It's for my ulcer." The pharmacist responds, "Yes, Zantac® is used in the treatment of ulcers."
   b. **Patient is unaware of indication:** Ms. Williams, "No, he (the doctor) just told me it would help me with my heartburn." The pharmacist responds, "Zantac® is a medication commonly used in the treatment of ulcers and excess stomach acid."
2. "HOW DID THE DOCTOR TELL YOU TO TAKE THE MEDICA-TION?"

a. **Patient is aware of medication regimen:** Ms. Williams responds, "The doctor told me to take it in the morning and before I go to bed at night." The pharmacist reviews the prescription label directions[11] with the patient and offers, "Good. It is important that you don't stop taking the medication unless the physician advises you otherwise. If you take a full course of therapy correctly, the chances that your ulcer will be gone are excellent."

b. **Patient is unaware of medication regimen:** Ms. Williams replies, "The doctor told me to take it twice a day but I don't know for how long." The pharmacist reviews the prescription label directions[11] with the patient and suggests, "You should take one tablet in the morning and the second one before you go to bed at night. Also, you should not stop taking the medication unless the physician advises you otherwise. If you take a full course of therapy correctly, the chances that your ulcer will be gone are excellent."

3. "WHAT DID THE DOCTOR TELL YOU ABOUT SIDE EFFECTS, INTERACTIONS, AND OTHER WARNINGS ABOUT THIS MEDICATION?"

a. **Patient is aware of side effects:** Ms. Williams responds, "The doctor told me there are few side effects but I may get a headache or some stomach upset. He (the doctor) told me rarely did the drug cause liver problems." The pharmacist replies, "That's correct, liver problems are rare. However, if you see any yellowing of the skin or eyes, or if your urine turns the color of cola you should contact your physician."

b. **Patient is unaware of side effects:** Ms. Williams responds, "The doctor just told me to call him if I had any problems and come back and see him in a month." The pharmacist offers, "There are a few minor side effects such as headache or stomach upset. Rarely, the medication may lead to liver problems. However, if your skin or eyes turn yellow, or if your urine turns the color of cola, you should contact your physician."

4. REFILL INFORMATION

"Ms. Williams there are two more refills on this prescription. This bottle should last one month. If the medication is working for you, the doctor will probably want you to continue on it for about two more months. Please come back then and I will be happy to refill it for you."

---

[11] Take one tablet by mouth twice daily in morning (9 a.m.) and at bedtime (11 p.m.) until told to stop for ulcer.